The ABC's of
Coronary Heart Disease

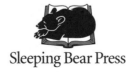

Sleeping Bear Press

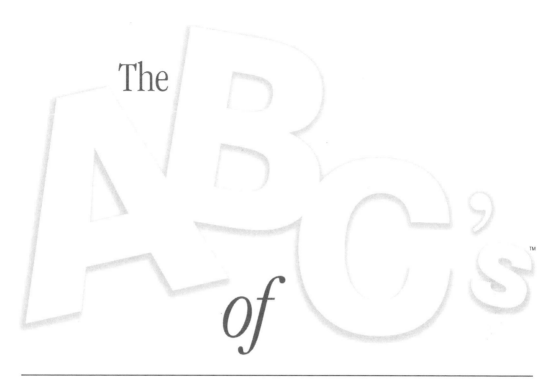

The ABC's *of* Coronary Heart Disease

By James J. Maciejko, M.S., Ph.D., F.A.C.C.
Director, Preventive Cardiology Program, Division of Cardiology,
St. John Hospital and Medical Center
Associate Professor, Department of Internal Medicine,
Wayne State University School of Medicine, Detroit, Michigan

Copyright © 2001 Sleeping Bear Press

Illustrations by Patrick J. Gloria

Sleeping Bear Press
310 North Main Street
P.O. Box 20
Chelsea, MI 48118
www.sleepingbearpress.com

Printed and bound in the United States.
10 9 8 7 6 5 4 3 2 1

Library of Congress Cataloging-in-Publication Data

Maciejko, James J.
The ABC's of coronary heart disease / James J. Maciejko.
p. cm.
Includes index.
ISBN 1-886947-99-6 (alk. Paper)
1. Coronary heart disease—Popular works. I. Title.
RC685.C6 M235 2001
616.1'23—dc21
    00-012249

Dedication

To Dr. George J. Grega, Dr. Bruce J. Kottke,
Dr. David R. Holmes, Dr. Melvyn Rubenfire,
Dr. Nicholas Z. Kerin, Dr. Robert J. Stomel—my
mentors, who through their guidance, allowed my
career to take the path that has led to this book.

Acknowledgments

I would like to thank Lynn Henning of the *Detroit News* who first approached me with the idea of writing a book on the most recent advances in the treatment of coronary heart disease and its link to cholesterol. His encouragement and insight have been greatly appreciated.

I would also like to thank my patients for posing the questions that have challenged me to critically evaluate the recent medical literature regarding the effective management of coronary heart disease. This information has become the basis of this book.

I express special gratitude to Amy Hockey, Anne Lewis, and Felicia Macheske at Sleeping Bear Press who have guided me through the book writing process and a special thank you to Patrick Gloria for illustrations which supplement the text and provide the reader with a better understanding of the concepts.

"What the reader learns and retains from *The ABC's of Coronary Heart Disease* is what is important, not what is often communicated or perceived through the media."

—Dr. James J. Maciejko

Preface

This book is written for the 14 million people who have been diagnosed with coronary heart disease. My intention is to assist in their understanding of this disease and what they can do to reduce their risk of further complications. The sequel to this book, *The ABC's of Preventing Coronary Heart Disease* is for the remaining people who have not been diagnosed, many of whom are at heightened risk for developing this disease, and will focus on the ways they can reduce their risk of acquiring coronary heart disease.

I have observed through my years of conducting clinical research trials in patients with coronary heart disease and in those who have been referred to me by their cardiologists to assist in reducing further complications, that many have a number of misconceptions regarding this disease and how it should be treated. I have also perceived that during my lectures to medical students, residents, and practicing physicians that they, too, have misconceptions.

This book's intent is to explain coronary heart disease in understandable terms and to identify and resolve the common misconceptions associated with it. **It will highlight the latest discoveries and breakthrough treatments of the past three years for this disease. It is this new information that has dramatically changed the approach to managing coronary heart disease patients.** You may find that the information in this book somewhat contradicts traditional concepts and beliefs about coronary heart disease. Yet new discoveries bring about change that is beneficial.

Only through understanding this disease and its treatment will this epidemic that exists today—not only in the United States but in all westernized countries—be reduced. Successfully doing this really does rest in the hands of those who have this disease. Believe it or not, you—the patient—ultimately drive the ways and means by which your illnesses and maladies are treated. By understanding coronary heart disease and learning the most effective methods for treating it, you will help determine the pace and outcome of the medical profession's quest to reduce its prevalence and devastation.

Foreword

Coronary heart disease and atherosclerosis of the major blood vessels are the leading causes of death and disability in the western world. Despite the significance of these diseases and increased public awareness there remains considerable confusion among patients and, unfortunately, many physicians. As a result of this confusion, the number of disabilities and deaths from coronary heart disease remains higher than necessary.

Dr. Maciejko's emphasis on reducing cardiovascular risk through diet, exercise and/or drugs in order to lower cholesterol is important to anyone who has been diagnosed with coronary heart disease or atherosclerosis. It is especially important if bypass graft surgery, balloon dilation or coronary stent placement is being contemplated as treatment. There is all too often the impression that fixing the vessel through the use of one of these procedures "fixes the problem." While these procedures represent some of the most important advances in treating coronary heart disease, they provide, as pointed out by Dr. Maciejko, mainly symptomatic relief without altering the underlying risk of a future heart attack or cardiovascular event. Exceptions to the use of these procedures is for those with severe disease such as narrowing of the left main coronary artery or severe narrowing of all three major coronary arteries.

The most effective means of preventing a heart attack and future cardiovascular events in a patient with known coronary heart disease, whether or not they undergo any of the above mentioned surgical procedures, is to prevent insignificant coronary lesions (less than 50% diameter constriction) from eroding or rupturing. Once a lesion has ruptured it completely occludes blood flow to the heart muscle by clot formation. Lowering blood cholesterol, in particular LDL-cholesterol, in conjunction with lifestyle changes and medicines (aspirin, beta-blockers and possibly angiotensin-converting enzyme inhibitors), are the most effective measures for the prevention of a heart attack. In many cases, aggressive lipid reduction through diet and/or drugs may also reduce the symptoms of coronary artery disease and prevent the need for balloon dilation or coronary stent placement.

The increased understanding provided by *The ABC's of Coronary Heart Disease* goes a long way toward dispelling many of the misconceptions about coronary heart disease. It is essential reading for anyone diagnosed with or caring for someone with coronary heart disease. The knowledge gained from this book will allow a patient to more fully understand their illness and provide the opportunity to have a more informed dialogue with their physician. The end results, I believe, will be better long-term compliance to medical therapy and increased prevention of disability and death related to coronary heart disease.

—Bertram Pitt, M.D.

Understanding Coronary Heart Disease

Treatment of Coronary Heart Disease and Common Misconceptions

Taking Responsibility for Your Cardiovascular Health

Introduction

The ABC's of Coronary Heart Disease was written primarily for the 14 million Americans who currently have been diagnosed with coronary heart disease. It is actually estimated that several million additional Americans (it is believed that the number could be between 25 and 50 million) have the disease but have not yet been diagnosed. If you are one of them, think you may be one of them, or know one of them, this book should be of considerable interest. If, at first glance, it all seems a bit overwhelming, then make sure you read this Introduction in its entirety. It will help you absorb all of the primary messages of this book and hopefully allow you to feel much better informed and far less intimidated by what unfolds as you confront this silent, insidious disease.

The information in The ABC's of Coronary Heart Disease is different than the information in the majority of books currently available on the subjects of heart disease and cholesterol. This book was written based on the latest information reported in the leading medical journals and on the six most common misconceptions that people have about these medical issues. These misconceptions are consequential because they often lead to less than optimal treatment of the disease, and lack of the most prudent initiatives to reduce risk of further complications of coronary heart disease.

The Six Common Misconceptions about Coronary Heart Disease

▶ Heart bypass surgery and angioplasty cure, or partially cure, coronary heart disease.

▶ The severity or extent of the cholesterol blockages in the coronary arteries is a good indicator of the likelihood of a heart attack.

▶ Cardiovascular disease is primarily a man's disease.

▶ The only benefit of cholesterol-lowering medicines is reducing the blood cholesterol level.

▶ Cholesterol-lowering medicines (statins) are associated with serious side effects.

▶ Only high cholesterol levels are linked to coronary heart disease and heart attack.

Coronary heart disease is the most common form of cardiovascular disease, which collectively, are diseases of the heart and blood vessels and are responsible for about half of all deaths in the United States. According to the 1998 Heart and Stroke statistical update by the American Heart Association, 961,000 people (over 456,000 males [47%] and about 506,000 [53%] females) in the United States died from cardiovascular diseases, accounting for one of every two deaths and making them the leading cause of death and disability in this country. Actually, more than one in five males and females have some form of diagnosed cardiovascular disease.

These 1998 statistics indicate that you are two times more likely to die from a form of cardiovascular disease than from any form of cancer, which claimed 282,000 males and 257,000 females in that same year. In fact, according to the most recent National Center for Health Statistics computations, **if all forms of cardiovascular disease were eliminated, life expectancy would increase by ten years. On the other hand, if all forms of cancer were eliminated, life expectancy would increase by only three years**.

These statistics are particularly relevant to women. Women are at much higher risk and are more likely to die from diseases of the heart and blood vessels than from any form of cancer. There is no better time for women to accept how important it is to understand cardiovascular disease and take preventive measures against it in the same manner they have diligently acknowledged their vulnerability to cancer over the past decade.

To emphasize this point, surveys indicate that most women are far more concerned about breast cancer than cardiovascular disease, yet only one in 26 women will succumb to breast cancer while one in two will die from cardiovascular disease. Breast cancer is certainly a devastating disease; however, if women do not also understand their risk of cardiovascular disease they may not take the necessary steps to reduce their risk, thereby increasing their prospects of living a full and healthy life.

Since 1984, in terms of total numbers of deaths, cardiovascular disease claimed the lives of more women than men and the gap continues to widen. The harsh reality is that cardiovascular diseases are the number one killers of women, claiming more than one-half million females every year. That is more lives than are claimed by the next 16 leading causes of death in women combined. Furthermore, within six years after having a heart attack, 23% of women who survived will have another.

This information is not common knowledge largely because the print, radio, and television media's coverage of health issues is generally directed at non-cardiovascular diseases, such as cancer and AIDS. Nonetheless, since 1900, cardiovascular diseases have been the number one killer in the United States in every year except 1918. In that year, infections, including tuberculosis, diphtheria, influenza, and measles were the leading causes of death. Today, even in the third world countries where infectious diseases are still the leading causes of death, cardiovascular disease mortality is increasing.

Figure 1 compares the percentage of deaths from cardiovascular disease to percentages of other major causes of death in the United States.

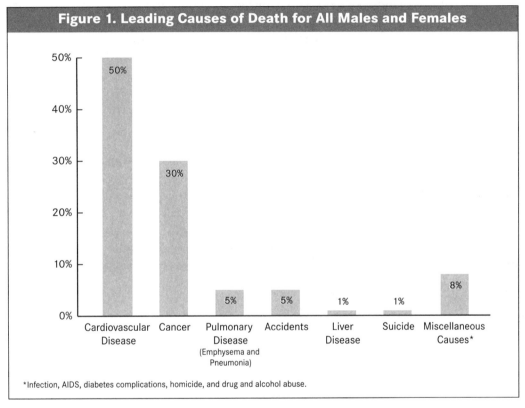

Figure 1. Leading Causes of Death for All Males and Females

*Infection, AIDS, diabetes complications, homicide, and drug and alcohol abuse.

Despite advances in treatment, which are helping to save some lives, cardiovascular diseases in our country are at epidemic proportions and have placed a huge economic burden on society. A major reason is that the number of people living with cardiovascular disease is increasing exponentially and so is the cost of treating them. It is not surprising then, that the United States spends more on care for cardiovascular diseases than on any other disease category. With a 5% annual increase added to actual 1994 figures, the estimated total annual medical bill of our nation is currently over $750 billion. Of that amount, it is estimated that the total costs for all cardiovascular diseases are over $290 billion per year.

That dollar amount represents the sum of both direct costs (every dollar that is spent on cardiovascular health care) and indirect costs (every expense incurred by all involved parties throughout a disease or illness). Direct costs are those expenses that are tallied from both public health care providers—Medicare and Medicaid—and private health care providers such as Blue Cross/Blue Shield, managed care organizations (HMOs) and medical insurance companies—as well as individual out of pocket expenses. Indirect costs are the total dollars spent or lost as a result of the diagnosis, treatment and recovery from a cardiovascular disease. These include every cost and expense—from loss of work and productivity to gas and maintenance on your vehicle during your commute to and from the doctor or hospital and the expense incurred by your employer to replace you during your illness and recovery period. Therefore, it only stands to reason that if we put forth an effort to reduce the magnitude of the cardiovascular disease epidemic, we would all save considerable money.

The most common form of cardiovascular disease is coronary heart disease. Coronary heart disease constitutes about 60% of all cardiovascular disease in the United States *(Figure 2).*

About 14 million Americans have diagnosed coronary heart disease and over 500,000 die each year from it and its major complication—heart attack. Every 29 seconds an American will suffer a heart attack and every minute, someone will

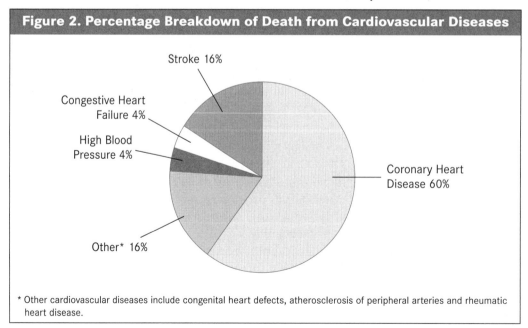

Figure 2. Percentage Breakdown of Death from Cardiovascular Diseases

Stroke 16%

Congestive Heart Failure 4%

High Blood Pressure 4%

Coronary Heart Disease 60%

Other* 16%

* Other cardiovascular diseases include congenital heart defects, atherosclerosis of peripheral arteries and rheumatic heart disease.

die from one. This year (2001) an estimated 1,100,000 Americans will have had a new or recurrent heart attack and about one-third to one-half will die from them. In addition, about 9% of men and 18% of women will suffer a stroke (complete stoppage of blood through one of the arteries in the brain) within five years after having a heart attack. Over 250,000 people die each year from "sudden death," which is death within one hour of the onset of a heart attack and is caused because the heart fibrillates or quivers as a result of the heart attack. A quivering heart does not pump blood effectively.

Worldwide, coronary heart disease and its major expression, heart attack, are the highest in Finland, Scotland, England, Hungary, and India, where almost 600 of every 1,000 male deaths are related to coronary heart disease. Japan, with less than 75 per 1,000, has one of the lowest death rates in the world from coronary heart disease. The United States is in between with approximately 400 deaths per 1,000 caused by coronary heart disease.

Age, gender, and race significantly impact an individual's risk of developing coronary heart disease. Of those three risk factors, advancing age is certainly the most significant. Eighty-five percent of the people who die of coronary heart disease are 65 years or older. Age is not a modifiable risk factor and therefore, it is critical that those who are in their sixth and seventh decades of life become aware of how aging is associated with increased risk of coronary heart disease. Seniors must speak with their doctors to learn how to reduce their risk through modifying the factors that are within their control.

Of those working adults under 65 who suffer and survive their initial heart attack, about 90% are able to return to work. However, two-thirds of them do not make a full recovery. In other words, even though they are able to resume their employment, they may not be able to do everything they once could, such as playing tennis, jogging or walking an 18-hole golf course.

About 48% of men and 63% of women who died suddenly from a heart attack had no prior symptoms or knowledge that they had the disease. About 40% of men die from their first heart attack, whereas 50% of women die from their first heart attack. Death rates from coronary heart disease are about 7% higher for black males than white males and 35% higher for black females than white females.

The purpose of the aforementioned facts and statistics is not to fill your mind with numbers and percentages or instill fear; rather it is to inform you of the enormous ramifications of this disease. They are certainly sobering statistics, and are necessary to demonstrate the serious implications of cardiovascular diseases, and coronary heart disease in particular.

Before proceeding further, it is necessary for you to know what coronary heart disease is. It will be explained in greater detail in Chapter 2, but at this point, you should know that it is the disease of the heart muscle or myocardium, caused by the stoppage of blood flow through a coronary artery that supplies the heart muscle with the oxygen and nutrients contained in the blood. The coronary arteries (there are two, a right and a left), which carry the blood to the heart muscle, may become partially or completely blocked by cholesterol (fat) deposits in the inner lining *(Figure 3)*. These cholesterol

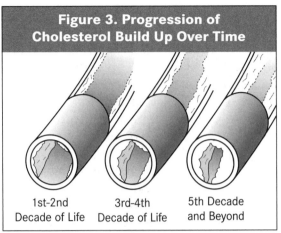

Figure 3. Progression of Cholesterol Build Up Over Time

1st-2nd Decade of Life   3rd-4th Decade of Life   5th Decade and Beyond

deposits, also called plaques, are referred to in medical terms as atherosclerosis (hardening of the arteries). When a coronary artery is encumbered with cholesterol deposits or plaques, it is termed coronary artery disease. Coronary artery disease, if significant enough to completely block the artery and stop the flow of blood (which is a heart attack), can cause coronary heart disease (death of the heart muscle or portion of it due to the lack of blood). **It is my hope that while the terms coronary artery disease and coronary heart disease are often used interchangeably, this explanation clarifies the subtle difference.**

A variety of genetic or inherited factors, as well as environmental influences such as diet, body weight, and smoking habits, certainly relate to the prevalence of coronary heart disease culturally and individually. However, the single most effective way to reduce the risk of developing coronary artery disease or having a heart attack is by aggressively lowering your cholesterol level, specifically the so-called bad cholesterol, or LDL (low density lipoprotein)-cholesterol. This has consistently proved to be true in controlled interventional studies, not only in individuals with coronary heart disease (those who have had a heart attack or heart surgery), but also in those without the disease. Results from controlled interventional studies largely establish how medicine should be practiced. This is referred to as "evidence-based medicine."

A slight detour from our discussion about cholesterol and coronary heart disease is warranted at this point. Your first impression of the following discussion about how the medical profession conducts research studies may be that it seems out of place in a book focusing on the most likely cause of your death. However, it is important, and you will soon appreciate its significance as you continue your journey through these pages.

Perhaps you've been confused by the conflicting results of medical studies that are reported. One day the newspaper prints a story claiming that a research study has indicated that drinking coffee is not harmful, and then a few weeks later another story about a recent study indicates that it is. This has also happened with a variety of other things such as garlic supplements, vitamins C and E, alcohol, fiber, and types and extent of exercise.

These mixed messages are frustrating and make it very difficult to know what you can do to attempt to improve your health, and reduce your risk of acquiring a disease or becoming ill. To better interpret the results of a reported research study, it is important to understand the category or type of medical research study. There are basically two types of medical studies, survey and interventional. The majority of research studies are of the survey type. Only a small portion of medical research studies is of the interventional type.

The primary goal of survey studies or observational studies is to identify an association between specific characteristics from a large group of people and the development of a particular outcome such as cancer or heart disease. People participating in a survey study are followed for a period of time (usually several years) and several characteristics, such as weight, diet, smoking habits, exercise patterns, or gender are compared in those participants who develop a disease versus those that remain free of the disease. An association between a characteristic or trait (called a variable) and the disease (called the outcome) can be identified. Any association that is observed in a survey study between a particular variable and an outcome, even a very strong association, *does not prove cause and effect.* The results obtained from survey studies are pertinent only to the group of people participating in the study and the particular time the study was carried out. Therefore, results may differ from one survey study to another. The associations identified from survey studies are useful for generating hypotheses or a tentative assumption about what may be causing a particular disease or disorder. The results by no means indicate that a variable caused the outcome. Therefore, results of a survey study do not indicate that you should change your lifestyle of healthy habits.

Results of survey studies examining the same issues can, and often do, give variable results. That is because little, if any, control of the participants is involved. A lack of control may give different results that arise from any number of non-controlled issues including geographic locations, populations, ages, genders and social and genetic factors that vary from one group of study participants to another.

As pointed out, the true purpose for conducting a survey study is to generate trends leading to the establishment of hypotheses or postulates that can be tested for validity in an interventional study. **The highest standard of evidence for cause and effect is obtained from the interventional study.** These are studies where a particular intervention, such as a drug, specific diet or nutritional supplement, or a specific exercise program, is given to one group of the study participants while the other group, considered the "control group," receives a placebo (sugar pill, standard diet, or no exercise beyond one's normal routine activity). The two groups (or more if several interventions are being evaluated) of participants will be the same or controlled relative to age, gender, weight, racial mix, and social habits (e.g., smoking, the use of alcohol, diet, etc.). The groups of participants are identical in almost all ways, except that some will receive an active intervention while the others receive an inactive or placebo intervention. The impact of the intervention on the outcome is determined. The results of an interventional study are relevant and do form the basis for treating disease and making recommendations about improving one's health. Therefore, if you are confused about the results of a medical study, try to determine if it is an observational (survey) or interventional study. If the results are from a survey study, do not overreact because a hypothesis is the only point that can be made of the results. If the results are from an interventional study, place more credibility in the findings, and discuss with your doctor whether they have relevance to you. Results from controlled, interventional studies will usually be similar.

It is through multiple interventional studies that lowering the bad cholesterol portion of the total blood cholesterol (i.e., LDL) has shown to significantly reduce the chance of heart attack, death, stroke, and hospitalizations for coronary heart disease. Lowering your blood level of bad cholesterol prevents it from depositing in the lining of the arteries thereby causing coronary artery disease. Even if you already have cholesterol deposits, lowering the LDL-cholesterol will stabilize these plaques and make them less likely to cause a heart attack. Essentially, reducing bad cholesterol (LDL) "cures" a portion of coronary arterial cholesterol deposits (i.e., atherosclerosis) in much the same way that an antibiotic "cures" an infection.

Traditionally, treatment of coronary artery disease has largely focused on alleviating its symptoms, such as shortness of breath, chest discomfort and fatigue. Surgical procedures, including coronary artery bypass grafting surgery (heart bypass surgery) and percutaneous transmural coronary angioplasty (angioplasty), and medicines such as nitrates and calcium-channel blockers, help increase blood flow through the partially blocked coronary arteries and reduce these symptoms and increase your exercise capacity. As a result, they make a patient feel better and improve one's quality of life. However, controlled, interventional studies of heart bypass surgery and angioplasty have shown that these surgical procedures do relatively little to reduce the chance or risk of a patient having a coronary event (i.e., fatal or nonfatal heart attack, unstable angina episode, or sudden death). Unfortunately, the majority of people believe the opposite.

The belief that heart bypass surgery substantially reduces the chances of having a heart attack received tremendous support in January of 2000 when David Letterman had heart bypass surgery. The story was widely publicized and the general impression given to the public was that David Letterman was prolonging his life and significantly reducing his chance of having a heart attack by having this surgery. In reality, this was probably not the case. Generally you are almost as likely to have a heart attack before heart bypass surgery as you are after the procedure. Only in an emergency situation, or when a blockage in a specific segment of the coronary artery (called the left main segment) is bypassed, or if three or more major coronary arteries are severely narrowed does this surgery *modestly* reduce the risk of further complications including death. For example, if you are in the midst of having a heart attack and arrive at the hospital almost immediately, your chance of survival will significantly improve if you have heart bypass surgery. The same applies to angioplasty. This procedure, like heart bypass surgery, has little to no impact on reducing one's risk of having a heart attack or coronary event. Again, only in the emergency situation will angioplasty potentially save a life. However, the majority of these surgical procedures are not performed in the emergency situation. Rather, they are conducted as elective procedures scheduled several days or weeks in advance.

By no means do I intend to imply that heart bypass surgery and angioplasty are not important or useful. They do reduce the symptoms of coronary artery disease (i.e., they will likely make you feel better) and therefore improve the quality of life. However, do not confuse relief of symptoms with improving your chances of not having a heart attack or dying from coronary artery disease complications (i.e., sudden death). In Chapter 4, I address in detail the six common misconceptions about coronary heart disease and its treatment that were listed on page 13. If you have been diagnosed with coronary heart disease, dispel these misconceptions, become a better-educated health care consumer and discuss the treatment issues with your cardiologist or physician. You will be "stacking the deck in your favor" toward improving your chances of having a better quality of life.

Before proceeding further, I would like to clarify what risk means in the context of increasing or decreasing your chances of acquiring coronary artery disease or having or dying from a heart attack. I will borrow an analogy from Dr. Alan S. Brown. Dr. Brown, a well-known cardiologist in Naperville, Illinois explains risk to his patients by pointing out the difference between crossing the street on a red light or a green light. If you have risk factors for coronary heart disease (such as high cholesterol, a smoking habit, high blood pressure, diabetes, or excess weight) you're crossing the street on a red light. We all know that the risk of getting hit by a car in this situation is quite high. However, there is a possibility, although small, that you can get across the street without being hit.

We also know that if the light were green, you'd have a better chance of getting across the street safely. Simply put, if you go through life with risk factors, you're crossing the street on a red light and your risk of developing coronary heart disease, or having a coronary event, is high. However, if you adapt measures to reduce your risk, it is similar to switching the red light to a green light, and thereby reducing your risk of having coronary heart disease.

It is very clear that many Americans are crossing the street on a red light when it comes to coronary heart disease and its complications. This is contrary to the notion that good health is everyone's fundamental priority. Few would argue with the adage "everything else in life is secondary to good health." Yet it seems we are shying away from the responsibility. We Americans must realize that we are far more accountable for our health status than our habits and behavior demonstrate. Our eating habits, activity level, sleeping habits and our use of alcohol and tobacco are all within our control and have a significant impact on our degree of health. **In short, while mortality (death) is inevitable, morbidity (sickness or illness) is preventable.**

While the primary reason for good health is to achieve and maintain a happy and richly fulfilled life, there is also another important reason. As mentioned earlier, health care costs in this country are rising exponentially. These rising costs have made it necessary for the government and private sectors to intervene in an attempt to control and reduce them. While these public and private health care providers assure us that controlling costs will not compromise the quality of health care delivered, we only need to read the newspapers and listen to the radio to recognize that this is not always the case. People can be denied health care coverage for tests or treatment by their health insurance provider that are considered necessary by their physician.

The common reasons given by health care insurers for denying payment include: lack of a referral by the primary care physician to a specialist; the test or treatment requested by their physician was not preapproved; alternative (usually less expensive and less effective) therapies are available; the necessity of the recommended treatment is questioned. Generally the reasons are designed to reduce costs and may not adequately take into account the medical need of the patient. Sometimes when physicians underutilize tests and therapies, they recoup the savings they have passed on to the provider. This appears to be an obvious conflict of interest. However, as long as controlling health care costs remains important, the debate as to how to best accomplish this will continue. In the meantime, the quality of your health care can no longer be assumed on your part.

You—the health care consumer—must accept how important it is to play an active role in maintaining your good health. You must learn to take responsibility for those aspects of your health that are within your control and make every effort to ensure, to the best of your ability, that the most appropriate tests and treatments available are being provided to you when necessary. You can learn to do this. First, it is important that you gain an understanding of the diseases and disorders that most threaten your health and then learn the specifics of those diseases that you have been, or may be, diagnosed with.

By staying knowledgeable, you will be able to interact at a higher level with your health care professionals and insurers. In the event that illness does strike, you will be better prepared to ask your doctor appropriate questions and actively participate in the recovery and maintenance processes. Basically, you will be more likely to receive the necessary and most suitable tests and therapies when, if ever, they are needed. Sitting back and trusting that your insurer will allow your doctor to provide you with the most appropriate health care is not necessarily the best approach in this ever-changing health care system. Nor is requesting a particular treatment or procedure that you mistakenly believe is in your best interest.

Controlling the coronary heart disease epidemic is a tremendous responsibility for health care professionals to carry alone. In order for them to be successful, there must be a shift in the focus of treatment for coronary heart disease to include not only the alleviation of symptoms but effective treatment of the underlying cause of this disease, i.e., atherosclerosis. It will ultimately be up to you, the consumer, to become knowledgeable about your heart and blood vessel health, and work with your physicians and other health-care professionals to achieve this goal. Essentially, you will need to take charge of your own health-care destiny to make sure you receive the utmost in proper coronary heart disease prevention and treatment.

It is for that reason I have written *The ABC's of Coronary Heart Disease*. My intention is to provide you with the knowledge and understanding necessary to "stack the deck in your favor" and reduce your chance of experiencing a coronary event—at any level—from minor to fatal. I am particularly interested in educating the 14 million Americans and their families who have already been diagnosed with coronary heart disease and are the highest risk group for heart attack, stroke, and sudden death, so that they too can "begin crossing the street on a green light."

A

Understanding Coronary Heart Disease

Chapter 1
Understanding the Cardiovascular System

In order to understand the risks, causes, and effective treatments for coronary heart disease, you must first learn about your cardiovascular system. As you begin reading this chapter, you may become intimidated or even frustrated by the technical nature of the anatomy (structure) and physiology (function) of your cardiovascular system. Nonetheless, in many cases there is really no other way to describe or define some of the structure and functions of the cardiovascular system without going into this level of detail. If you find yourself getting lost, don't be alarmed—there are doctors who don't fully understand these concepts. Therefore, if it becomes too challenging, simply move on to Chapter 2 or just review the illustrations and read the brief descriptions.

Essentially, the cardiovascular system's function is to pump and transport the life fluid (blood) throughout the body so that it can deliver oxygen and nutrients (such as glucose) to, and remove waste products (such as carbon dioxide and urea) from, all cells in the body.

The cardiovascular system is composed of a pump, the heart, and a series of tubes, or passageways, for transporting blood, which are the blood vessels. Your heart is approximately the size of your fist, and weighs about three-quarters of a pound. Blood vessels (tubes) are categorized as arteries, veins, and capillaries. Arteries transport blood from the heart to all tissues and organs in the body. Veins drain the blood from all tissues and organs and carry it back to the heart. Capillaries (located between the arteries and veins) permit the oxygen and nutrients in the blood to get to the cells of an organ and allow for the waste material to leave the cells and get into the blood so the veins can drain it away.

Remember:
- ▶ arteries transport the blood.
- ▶ veins drain the blood.
- ▶ capillaries facilitate the function of the cardiovascular system.

Blood feeds the cells, so it is called the life fluid of the human body. It is composed of red and white blood cells, plasma, which is a mixture of serum (mostly water and nutrients) and platelets, a collection of small disc-like clotting proteins that are important in order for blood to clot.

- water + salt + nutrients = serum
- serum + platelets = plasma
- plasma + red and white blood cells = blood

The red blood cells carry oxygen to the cells that form an organ or tissue while the white blood cells offer protection from disease. White blood cells are a major component of the body's immune system. The major categories of white blood cells are leukocytes, lymphocytes, and monocytes. Cells of the body (making up the tissues and organs) extract oxygen and nutrients (the vitamins, minerals, lipids or fat, carbohydrates or sugar, water, and protein contained in the food you eat) from the blood and emit or discharge waste products (carbon dioxide and urea) back into the blood. These processes occur at the level of the tiniest blood vessels, called capillaries, which contain tiny holes or pores that allow these transfers to occur. The lungs replace the carbon dioxide (waste product) with oxygen, while other waste products of cells are removed from the blood by the kidneys, which form urine containing these waste products.

Located in the chest cavity, the heart is a muscular organ that sits between the lungs. Like all organs, it is made up of millions of microscopic units called cells. Most of the cells that make up the heart are medically referred to as cardiac myocytes or muscle cells. While each cell is capable of carrying on most characteristics of life, they all work together to allow the heart to perform its function. In addition to the heart, other examples of organs that are comprised of millions of unique cells that allow an organ to function in a specific way include your kidneys, which filter and clean your blood, your lungs, which add oxygen and remove carbon dioxide from your blood, and your pancreas, which manufactures hormones (insulin and glucogon) and enzymes that allow you to digest the food you eat. Each of these organs is formed by millions of similar cells to allow the organ to perform its necessary function(s).

The cardiovascular system's overall function is to deliver oxygen and nutrients to the cells that comprise all tissues and organs in the body and remove waste products from the cells. This is accomplished through the transportation of blood.

The heart (pump) receives and pumps the blood through the blood vessels and is structurally composed of four chambers. Two of the chambers, called atria or auricles, are reservoirs for the blood. They receive blood from the veins, which drain blood from the body and the lungs. The other two chambers are called ventricles and are the actual blood pumping chambers of the heart. The ventricles receive blood from the two atria.

Functionally, the heart is divided into two halves, the right and left, which are each composed of an atrium and a ventricle. In other words, the right half is composed of the right atrium and right ventricle, and the left half is composed of the left atrium and left ventricle. The blood that is received into the right atrium has been drained from all tissues and organs of the body, except the lungs. The left atrium receives blood that has been enriched with oxygen from the lungs.

Let us now begin to understand how the blood flows (circulation) throughout the entire cardiovascular system (i.e., heart and blood vessels). We begin with the amount of blood (approximately 3 ounces) contained in the right atrium (heart chamber) during one heart cycle, or heartbeat. This blood is delivered to the right atrium via the superior and inferior vena cavae. These are the two largest veins in the body with which all of the other smaller veins ultimately connect *(Figure 4)*.

The superior vena cava and inferior vena cava act as the major conduits that receive blood from smaller veins that have drained blood from all tissues and organs in the body except the lungs. The superior vena cava collects the blood

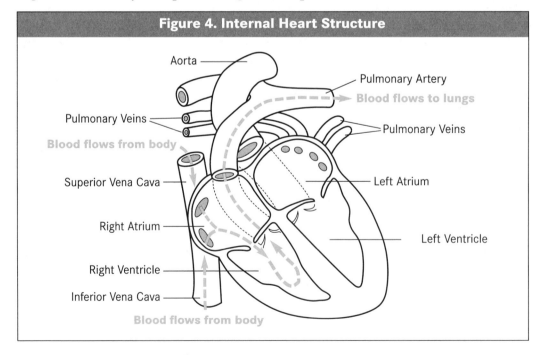

Figure 4. Internal Heart Structure

drained from the organs and tissues above the heart. The inferior vena cava collects the blood drained from the organs and tissues below the heart.

The right atrium deposits its blood into the right ventricle which pumps the blood into the lungs. The right atrioventricular (A/V) valve, or the tricuspid valve, separates the right atrium from the right ventricle. Only when this valve or door is opened will the blood from the right atrium be deposited into the right ventricle.

During a portion of the heartbeat, (called systole), the right ventricle will squeeze, which closes the tricuspid valve and opens the pulmonary valve. The pulmonary valve is located at the entrance to the pulmonary artery from the right ventricle. Blood is then ejected into this blood vessel (pulmonary artery). Since the tricuspid valve is closed, no blood will be pushed back into the right atrium when the right ventricle squeezes or contracts. When pumped into the pulmonary artery, the blood is delivered to the lungs where the carbon dioxide is removed and oxygen is added. The blood then drains from the lungs into the pulmonary veins.

The pulmonary veins deposit the blood into the left atrium of the heart. As with the right side of the heart, the left atrium is separated from the left ventricle by the left A/V valve, commonly known as the mitral valve. As this valve or door opens, the blood in the left atrium flows into the left ventricle. *(Figure 5)*.

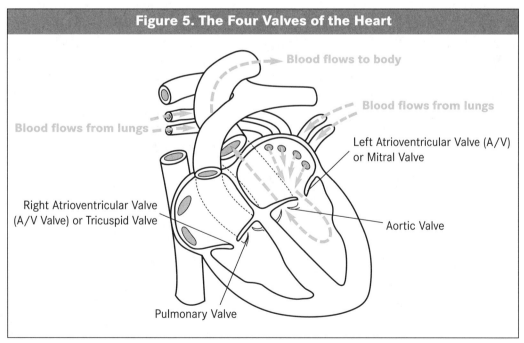

Figure 5. The Four Valves of the Heart

Blood flows to body

Blood flows from lungs

Blood flows from lungs

Left Atrioventricular Valve (A/V) or Mitral Valve

Right Atrioventricular Valve (A/V Valve) or Tricuspid Valve

Aortic Valve

Pulmonary Valve

During systole the left ventricle squeezes at the same instant the right ventricle squeezes. This squeezing, or contracting, of the left ventricle causes the mitral valve to close and the aortic valve to open and the blood is ejected into a single blood vessel called the aorta. The aortic valve is located at the entrance to the aorta from the left ventricle. The aorta is the largest artery in the body and transports blood to subsequently smaller arteries, such as the coronary arteries, so that blood and its nutrients can be delivered to all tissues and organs.

Once blood is squeezed from either the right ventricle into the pulmonary artery or from the left ventricle into the aorta, it cannot flow back into the ventricles because the pulmonary and aortic valves snap shut when the ventricles relax. When the ventricles relax, the right and left A/V valves (tricuspid and mitral) open and allow blood to move from the two atria into their respective ventricles. This coordinated opening and closing of the heart valves allows for the unidirectional flow of blood. In other words, heart valves function like one-way doors, allowing blood to move in only one direction and preventing it from backing up into the chamber from which it came.

The contraction (systole) and relaxation (diastole) of the right and left ventricles (heartbeat or cycle) must be synchronized for the entire cardiovascular system to work effectively. In a normal person who is at rest, the amount of blood pumped simultaneously by each ventricle of the heart is about six quarts per minute. (Three ounces per beat; 70 beats per minute; 3 x 70 = 210 ounces per minute, or 210/32* = 6 quarts per minute. *32 ounces in a quart.) During heavy work or exercise, the volume can increase to as much as 30 quarts per minute.

In order for the heartbeat to be coordinated, a series of electrical impulses are transmitted throughout the heart that allow for the appropriate contraction and relaxation to occur. A small group of cells allow for the impulse conduction or movement, and are essentially the power source and electrical system of the heart. These cells initiate an electrical impulse that conducts throughout the heart, leading to a coordinated heartbeat. These cells are similar to nerve cells like those in the brain and spinal cord. They form what is called the electrical conducting system of the heart *(Figure 6)*.

The electrical conducting system of the heart is comprised of three general components:
► the sinoatrial (SA) node
► the atrioventricular (AV) node
► and the His-Purkinje fibers.

The SA node is oval shaped and composed of a group of specialized heart cells that initiate the heartbeat signal. The SA node is known as the heart's primary pacemaker. It sets the rate of the heartbeat and is located at the top of the right atrium. The wave of electrical activity passes from the SA node through the right atrium to the AV node, which is the heart's secondary pacemaker.

The AV node is located at the bottom of the right atrium. At the AV node the impulse slows down slightly and then spreads to a specialized series of cells in the right and left ventricles which form the His-Purkinje fibers.

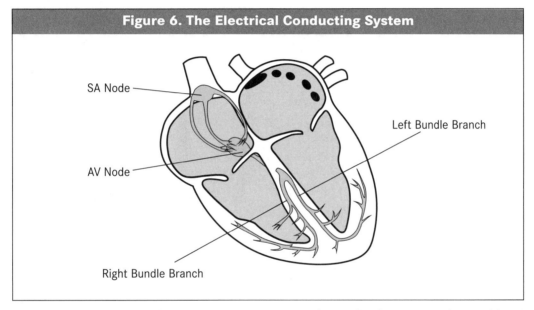

Figure 6. The Electrical Conducting System

SA Node

Left Bundle Branch

AV Node

Right Bundle Branch

This distribution of the electrical impulse through the His-Purkinje fibers triggers the contraction of the heart. While at a state of rest, the SA node triggers an impulse about 70 times per minute, which prompts about 70 heartbeats per minute.

To evaluate the electrical impulse and its movement through the heart, doctors use the electrocardiogram (EKG). An EKG shows the electrical activity that occurs in the heart and provides the doctor with information about heartbeats that may be too rapid (tachycardia), too slow (bradycardia), or irregular. A more complete description and actual tracing of an EKG is given in Chapter 3.

Because the heart is a muscular organ that pumps blood, it requires oxygen and nutrients to function properly. Most people think that the heart muscle (myocardium) is provided with the oxygen and nutrients it requires from the blood that fills the various chambers of the heart. This is not true. The coronary arteries supply the majority of the blood that provides the oxygen and nutrients needed by the heart muscle. Coronary arteries originate from two small openings or holes in the aorta called the coronary ostia. They are the first artery branches from the aorta *(Figure 7)*.

The right and left coronary arteries are two small arteries located on the surface of the heart and branch into numerous smaller arteries that penetrate into the heart muscle and provide oxygenated and nutritive blood to most of the cells making up the heart. The right and left coronary arteries and their main

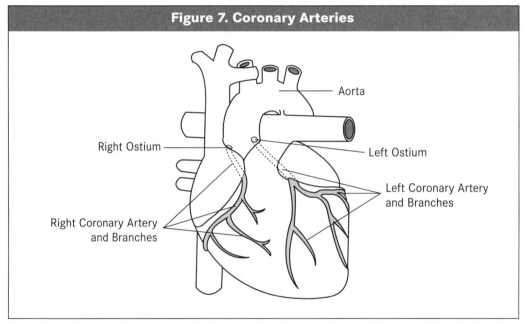

Figure 7. Coronary Arteries

Aorta

Right Ostium

Left Ostium

Left Coronary Artery and Branches

Right Coronary Artery and Branches

branches have a diameter of about 1/4 of an inch or 4-6 mm. Blood that has delivered its oxygen and nutrients to the heart muscle drains into a variety of small heart veins, which ultimately empty into the coronary sinus. The coronary sinus is the largest vein that receives blood from the heart muscle and deposits blood directly into the right atrium of the heart.

We have referred several times to the process of delivering oxygen and nutrients to the cells of the heart, as well as cells of all organs and tissues in the body. It is interesting to understand how this process occurs. Capillaries have been introduced in our discussion of the cardiovascular system and are key to delivering oxygen and nutrients to cells. Capillaries are the tiniest blood vessels contained in every tissue and organ of the body. They are the blood vessels located between the arteries and veins. These microscopic tubes contain tiny holes, called pores. Blood enters the capillaries from tiny arteries and exits from the capillaries into tiny veins or venules. Oxygen and nutrients leave the blood through the pores of the capillaries and enter into nearby cells. Likewise, it is through the pores that the waste products produced by the cells, such as carbon dioxide, enter into the blood. The pores are small enough so that red and white blood cells cannot pass through them. The capillaries in the lungs perform a vital function for the cardiovascular system. They allow for carbon dioxide to leave the blood and oxygen to enter the blood.

About 10% of the blood plasma (fluid without red and white blood cells) that escapes from the capillaries through the pores is not returned back to the capillaries. This escaped plasma penetrates in between cells and needs to be drained away so that it doesn't accumulate. A second circulation, called the lymphatic system, carries out the process of draining this excess fluid.

The lymphatic system can be thought of as the secondary cardiovascular system. However, it does not contain a pump or heart like the primary cardiovascular system. It contains only a series of tubes (called lymphatic vessels) and capillaries, and filters, called lymph nodes. Lymph nodes filter impurities from the collected fluid or lymph. They act as sieves to remove contaminants, such as bacteria and cellular debris, from the lymphatic fluid. They also contain specific white blood cells called lymphocytes. Lymphocytes destroy bacteria and viruses and help prevent the spread of infection and disease.

The tiniest lymphatic vessels are lymph capillaries. Just as those in the primary cardiovascular system, they also have tiny holes or pores. The small amount of plasma that escapes from the primary cardiovascular capillaries (about 10%) flows into the lymphatic capillaries through these pores. This fluid is now referred to as lymph.

As the lymph flows through the lymphatic capillaries, vessels, and nodes, it enters into progressively larger and larger lymphatic vessels. These large lymphatic vessels all converge into the largest lymphatic vessel in the body, called the thoracic duct. The thoracic duct connects to a large vein in the neck region of the body and allows for lymph to enter back into the blood.

If the lymphatic system is not functioning properly, the small amount of fluid or plasma that leaves the capillaries would remain in the tissue, leading to swelling. Medically, the terminology for this excess fluid is edema.

It will be easier for you to understand your cardiovascular system and how and why you should maintain it by remembering that it is responsible for pumping the life fluid (or blood) throughout your body. In summary, it is composed of the heart (pump) and blood vessels (tubes). Your heart is actually one large pump made up of two (right and left) smaller pumps, which are each composed of an atrium and a ventricle. The blood vessels, which are arteries, veins, or capillaries, deliver blood rich in oxygen and nutrients and remove blood containing waste products and carbon dioxide from all the cells and tissues of your body.

Your right atrium receives and collects blood from the body and deposits it into the right ventricle. Your right ventricle then pumps the blood into the lungs so oxygen can be added to and carbon dioxide removed from it. You provide your lungs with oxygen through inhaling and remove the carbon dioxide through exhaling. Your left atrium then receives the oxygen-enriched blood back from the lungs and delivers it to the left ventricle which pumps it into the aorta. The aorta branches into progressively smaller arteries that carry blood to all tissues and organs in the body except the lungs. The majority of the oxygen and nutrients required by your heart is supplied from the blood that is carried in your coronary arteries.

All cardiovascular diseases and maladies are related in one way or another to abnormal functioning of the heart and/or blood vessels. In Chapter 2, the variety of ways in which the cardiovascular system can malfunction will be discussed.

Chapter 2
Cardiovascular Diseases

There are a variety of types of cardiovascular diseases or disorders. It is important that you understand their differences so that the unique aspects of coronary heart disease will become more apparent to you. Upon understanding the brief descriptions of the various types of cardiovascular disease, you will be able to relate coronary heart disease to other forms of cardiovascular diseases and engage in a much more intelligent and productive conversation with your doctor and other health care professionals. This will also be especially useful if you are speaking to a friend or relative. For instance, if someone you know mentions that he or she has heart failure, you will immediately understand that it is probably not coronary heart disease and will not likely cause heart attacks. The purpose of this chapter then, is to provide you with a working knowledge to distinguish the differences between cardiovascular diseases or disorders and help clear up the confusion surrounding heart failure, valvular diseases, irregular heartbeats, and coronary heart disease. The intent is not to educate the reader comprehensively on all of the forms of cardiovascular disease. Rather, it is to provide a very general overview so that the distinction between coronary heart disease and other cardiovascular diseases is evident.

The Three Types

Diseases of the cardiovascular system (the heart and blood vessels) can be categorized into three types:

- mechanical defects
- electrical defects
- plumbing defects

Mechanical defects involve the heart and are those which lead to either reduced contraction and relaxation of the heart muscle (i.e., pumping capability), or improper closing and opening of the heart valves. Mechanical defects involve the heart or valves and result in the deficient pumping of blood throughout the blood vessels. Electrical defects involve the heart and cause irregularities (arrhythmias) in the heartbeat and, therefore, ineffective pumping of blood into the blood vessels. The final category, plumbing defects, are those that occur only in the blood vessels, generally the arteries, and are caused by the buildup of cholesterol in the inner lining of the artery, leading to the decreased flow of blood.

Mechanical Defects

Mechanical defects of the heart result in either the reduced pumping action of the heart or the defective opening and closing of the heart valves that separate the chambers of the heart and control the direction of blood flow.

Sick or diseased ventricles (pumping chambers of the heart) cause deficient pumping of blood by the heart. It is commonly referred to as heart failure. Heart failure can have several causes. Among them are:

1. defects in the heart muscle (myocardium) present at birth (congenital heart disease),
2. high blood pressure (hypertension),
3. primary disease of the heart muscle itself (idiopathic cardiomyopathy),
4. previous heart attack which killed off a portion of the heart muscle and compromises the heart's pumping action,
5. rheumatic fever.

Each one of these causes can reduce the strength of the pumping action of the heart, fill the heart chambers (ventricles) with too much blood, or limit the amount of blood entering into the heart chambers. The consequence of any of these occurrences is a reduced amount of blood pumped by the heart. When the heart does not pump appropriate amounts of blood to supply the oxygen needs of the body, a progressive series of signs and symptoms grouped under the category of congestive heart failure are triggered.

People with mild heart failure may show no significant signs or symptoms while at rest. However, their ability to perform exercise may be impaired. They will tire easily and experience shortness of breath (called dyspnea) because there is an inadequate supply of blood to the skeletal muscles and other organs of the body. In more significant cases of heart failure, blood flow is so reduced, due to the inadequate pumping of blood by the heart, that a patient can become bedridden, and swelling of the legs, ankles, and feet can occur. Fluid can also accumulate in the lungs (pulmonary edema) making breathing difficult. Ultimately, the cardiac output, or amount of blood pumped by the ventricles per heartbeat (remember, normal is about six quarts per minute during rest) may become too low to support life.

As indicated, a common feature of significant heart failure is the accumulation of tissue fluid or plasma in the legs, ankles, and feet. This swelling is referred to as edema. When the heart's pumping activity is reduced, blood flow slows down throughout the entire circulatory system of the body. Blood that is being returned to the heart through the veins also slows down and begins to accumulate in the veins. This increases the pressure in the veins and back into the capillaries, and forces the fluid of the blood (plasma) to seep out of the capillaries into the surrounding tissues of the legs, ankles, and feet. The lymphatic system is not adequate to carrying away all of this excess fluid.

The most serious consequence of heart failure, however, is the excess fluid that accumulates in the lungs. Basically, this occurs when the left ventricle of the heart isn't pumping blood adequately and the blood backs up and accumulates in the blood vessels of the lungs. Referred to as pulmonary edema, this situation leads to shortness of breath and an inability to breathe properly. The veins and capillaries in the lungs become engorged with blood. This elevates the pressure in the veins and capillaries and causes increased movement of blood fluid (plasma) out of the capillaries into the surrounding lung tissue. It usually worsens at night, because during the day, when an individual is in the upright posture, fluid accumulates in the legs. At night, when he or she is lying down, the plasma volume expands in the upper body and more readily accumulates into the pulmonary (i.e., lung) circulation.

The approach to treating heart failure and its symptoms (i.e., congestive heart failure) generally involves eliminating or reducing the cause of the failing heart. It is important that careful identification of the underlying cause be identified so that appropriate treatment can be given. Heart failure is usually categorized according to the degree of severity of symptoms, where less severe heart failure may be treated with healthy diet and exercise recommendations, whereas more significant heart failure conditions require medical and possibly surgical treatment. The New York Heart Association classifications of heart failure include the following four categories:

Class I—Patients with heart failure, yet no significant shortness of breath or weakness and no limit on physical activity.

Class II—Patients with heart failure and some modest degree of shortness of breath, fatigue or chest discomfort that may occur individually or in combination with normal activity.

Class III—The aforementioned symptoms occur with less than normal activity and the patient will usually be limited in his/her activities.

Class IV—The most severe degree of heart failure. Symptoms appear at rest.

An example of how Class III heart failure due to hypertension (high blood pressure) may be treated, follows. Sustained high blood pressure imposes an excessive workload on the heart. The heart needs to work more strenuously to push blood into the aorta and the artery branches because the pressure in these blood vessels is elevated. This, over time, causes the walls of the heart to thicken (called ventricular hypertrophy) and the heart muscle to weaken. The diseased heart no longer can pump blood as effectively as it should. The first step in treating this type of heart failure due to high blood pressure is to lower the blood pressure.

This can be accomplished with drugs called vasodilators. These drugs relax arteries and increase their inner diameters allowing for more blood to flow through them. By increasing the inner diameters of arteries, pressure from the blood against the walls of the arteries is lowered. The lowered blood pressure reduces the workload on the heart, since the pressure (or resistance the heart must overcome) in the arteries is lowered. Vasodilators are the cornerstone of medical heart failure therapy. The best known vasodilators are the angiotensin-converting enzyme (ACE) inhibitors. Examples include quinapril, captopril, enalapril, lisinopril, fosinopril, and ramipril.

As a second step, the physician may attempt to strengthen the contraction of the heart muscle with drugs such as digitalis, dobutamine, amrinone, and milronone. Drugs that strengthen the contraction of the heart muscle are called inotropic agents.

Finally, the excess fluid that accumulates in the ankles, feet, and lungs can be, in part, eliminated by diuretics, or water pills, which increase the excretion of fluid by the kidneys. Examples of some diuretics include hydrochlorothiazide, furosemide, bumetanide, spironolactone, amiloride, and indapamide.

People with heart failure (no matter what the cause) should follow a diet that limits salt intake and controls or reduces their body weight. Too much salt causes fluid retention in the blood vessels, which increases the blood pressure and makes the heart work harder. The average American consumes six to 18 grams of salt per day or approximately one to three teaspoons. Our body only requires about one to two grams of salt per day. A low-salt diet (sometimes called a low-sodium diet) for a person with heart failure allows for no more than two to three grams of salt per day. A low-salt diet helps the diuretic medicine (i.e., water pill) to work better. If you are reading food labels that report salt content as sodium, multiply the grams of sodium by 2.5 to give you the grams of salt. Alternatively, divide the grams of salt by 2.5 to give grams of sodium. Therefore, a low-sodium diet for a heart failure patient would be about one to 1.5 grams of sodium per day (i.e., 3 grams of salt ÷2.5 = 1.2 grams of sodium). The point to keep in mind is that with the right treatment and adjustments in the salt intake level, people with heart failure will usually feel better.

The other major category of "mechanical" cardiovascular diseases are those related to abnormal heart valve function. Remember, the heart has four valves—tricuspid, pulmonary, mitral, and aortic. They function like one-way doors that keep the blood moving forward (unidirectional) through the heart's chambers.

During the relaxing phase of the heart (called diastole) the two A/V valves (tricuspid and mitral) are open, allowing blood to flow from the right and left atria to the respective right and left ventricles. During diastole the pulmonary and aortic valves are closed. When the ventricles of the heart squeeze (called systole) the tricuspid and mitral valves snap shut and the pulmonary and aortic valves open, allowing blood to flow into the pulmonary artery and aorta. This synchronized opening and closing of the valves during the relaxation/contraction cycle of the heart (i.e., heartbeat) prevents blood from flowing backward.

The most common valve disorder involves the mitral valve. This is the valve that separates the left atrium and left ventricle. This disorder is referred to as mitral valve prolapse. Generally, it is not serious. A prolapsed mitral valve flops back into the left atrium when it closes shut during systole. This causes some blood to flow backward into the left atrium when the left ventricle squeezes. Therefore, not all the blood is pumped into the aorta. People with mitral valve prolapse may experience heart palpitations (flutters or quivers), weakness, chest discomfort or difficulty with breathing, particularly in more severe cases. A few may develop significant mitral regurgitation or a surging backflow of blood into the left atrium. These people may be at increased risk of stroke because blood clots can form in the left atrium and travel from the heart into an artery of the brain and plug it up. This of course, stops the flow of blood to a portion of the brain, which leads to a stroke.

Sometimes, a prolapsed mitral valve tends to attract bacteria, causing an infection. It is therefore recommended that a person with mitral valve prolapse take an antibiotic before dental or surgical procedures. As noted, however, mitral valve prolapse is generally not a serious problem. However, in severe cases the mitral valve may require surgical repair or even replacement.

Other heart valves can also malfunction due to damage (e.g., from a heart attack) or disease (infections, including rheumatic fever). Damage to the aortic valve (valve separating the left ventricle and aorta) can cause reduced blood flow into the aorta and increase the workload of the heart. Over time this can result in heart failure (i.e., weakening of the heart muscle with subsequent reduced pumping action). Surgical treatment (replacement of the damaged aortic valve with a prosthetic valve) is usually recommended for significant aortic valve disease. Sometimes significant disease of both the mitral and aortic valves occur. Under these conditions, both valves may need to be surgically replaced.

Endocarditis is the infection of the inner lining of the heart chambers that is caused by bacteria and can damage the valves. This can prevent the valves from opening or closing properly. A patient with endocarditis is quite ill (weak, fatigued and nauseated) and can have a fever. The heartbeat is rapid (greater than 100 beats per minute) and the heart valves can be severely damaged in a relatively short period of time. Treatment with an appropriate antibiotic (i.e., a drug that destroys bacteria) is essential.

Mechanical malfunctioning of the heart, whether it be deficient pumping activity or improper valve performance, is largely treated with medicines. Quality of life can generally be improved, particularly in patients who also adhere to an appropriate diet and exercise program. In more severe cases of congestive heart failure, cardiac transplantation may be considered. Also, as previously noted, surgical repair or replacement of heart valves is an option in the most severe cases of valvular disease.

Electrical Defects

Electrical defects of the heart cause irregularity or loss of rhythm (i.e., coordination) of the heartbeat. This condition is referred to medically as cardiac arrhythmia. Irregular heartbeats or arrhythmias can be harmless in some cases or serious in others. The normal speeding up or slowing down of the heart rate in response to the body's demands for blood is normal. A rapid heart rate (greater than 100 beats per minute) is called tachycardia. A slower than normal heart rate (less than 50 beats per minute) is called bradycardia. These changes in heart rate are considered normal because the SA node is initiating impulses based on the oxygen requirements of the body. The more activity a person is engaged in (e.g., running, exercising, climbing stairs), the more blood-carrying-oxygen is required by the body and the more rapid the heart rate.

There are, however, a number of serious heart rhythm disturbances or uncoordinated slow or rapid heartbeats that can interrupt the normal contraction-relaxation cycle of the heart.

Some common electrical defects of the heart include:
- ventricular tachycardia
- heart block
- supraventricular tachycardia
- atrial fibrillation
- sick sinus syndrome

All make the heart pump ineffectively so that not enough blood reaches the brain and other vital organs. When blood flow in the body is inadequate a person may faint or have chest pain, or death may even occur.

Ventricular tachycardias are some of the most serious types of heartbeat irregularities. Ventricular tachycardia occurs when the heartbeat impulse originates in the ventricles of the heart and not the SA node. (Remember, the SA node is located at the top of the right atrium and is the heart's primary pacemaker). This leads to uncoordinated contractions of the ventricles relative to the atria and ineffective pumping of the blood. The most serious type of ventricular tachycardia is fibrillation, which is an erratic quivering of the ventricles with little to no blood being pumped into the aorta and pulmonary artery. It is a life-threatening situation that requires immediate emergency medical attention.

Heart block is a form of arrhythmia marked by a reduction or block of the advancement of the electrical impulse from the SA node to the AV node. This results in reduced frequency of heartbeats (or ventricular contractions) to various degrees. Complete heart block causes severe bradycardia (i.e., extremely slow heart rate) that can lead to loss of consciousness or even death.

Supraventricular tachycardia arises in the atria (upper reservoir heart chambers) of the heart and is generally not life-threatening. In this electrical defect the atria contract at rates higher than the ventricles. Most of these arrhythmias are more of a nuisance and do not require medical treatment.

A significant type of supraventricular tachycardia is atrial fibrillation or the uncontrolled, uncoordinated rapid contraction or quivering of the atria. Atrial fibrillation is the most common form of cardiac arrhythmia. About three to five percent of Americans have atrial fibrillation. It is observed most often in people over 65, and develops when a disturbance in the electrical signals causes the two atria (upper chambers of the heart) to quiver. This precludes a significant portion of the blood from being forced into the heart's pumping chambers or ventricles. The blood collects inside the atria, increasing the chance for blood clots to form, which can travel through the body and potentially block an artery of the brain.

Atrial fibrillation is treated with medicines called antiarrhythmic drugs. Examples of a few are:
► quinidine and procainamide (Class I)
► propranolol, sotalol, timolol, metoprolol, and atenolol (Class II—also called beta-blockers)
► amiodarone (Class III)

The precipitating factor, or cause, for the atrial fibrillation determines the type of medicine the physician prescribes. Because of the heightened risk of blood clot formation and potential stroke, patients with atrial fibrillation usually receive anti-coagulant drugs to prevent blood clot formation. An example of an anticoagulant drug or "blood thinner" is warfarin.

Sick sinus syndrome is an electrical defect of the heart caused by a malfunction of the SA node. There are several abnormalities that can adversely impact the origination and/or the transmission of the electrical impulse from the heart's primary pacemaker (i.e., SA node). These include a heart attack in the region of the SA node, which destroys part of the node and degeneration of the node due to aging or infection. People with this type of arrhythmia may experience more than one rhythm abnormality. The heart may beat very slowly at times and then beat quite rapidly at other times. The symptoms correlate with the rhythm disturbance and can include dizziness, fatigue, fainting, and confusion. Sick sinus syndrome is usually treated by surgically implanting a pacemaker, which is a device that stabilizes the heartbeat.

Patients with very serious, life-threatening electrical abnormalities may require an implantable cardioverter/defibrillator (ICD), which will dramatically improve their chances of survival. This device is inserted surgically (like a pacemaker). The ICD monitors the heartbeat continuously, and when it detects an abnormal heartbeat, will give off a small shock to return the heartbeat to normal.

Plumbing Defects

The most common form of cardiovascular disease and the primary focus of this book is the major disease that affects the "plumbing," or flow of blood through the blood vessels. Bear in mind, plumbing disease refers to defects in the tubes (blood vessels) not defects in the pump (heart). You can prepare yourself for this discussion by using the analogy of the plumbing in your home. For a moment, think of your blood vessels, primarily the arteries, as the pipes in your home. When your pipes are clogged from hair or other debris, water will drain either very slowly or stop altogether. This is exactly what happens when your arteries become clogged. Your clogged pipes (arteries), specifically the coronary, arteries will dramatically slow or even stop the flow of blood, which can damage your heart.

By far the most prevalent of these "plumbing" diseases is atherosclerosis, which results from cholesterol accumulating in the inner linings of arteries. This cholesterol accumulation results in various sizes of clogs or deposits in the arteries. The arteries that most often become clogged with cholesterol are those that deliver blood to the heart (coronary arteries), the brain (carotid and cerebrovascular arteries), and the legs (femoral and popliteal arteries). In other words, certain arteries in the body are more susceptible to cholesterol buildup than other arteries. Generally, the most common arteries where cholesterol deposits occur are the coronary arteries. As mentioned in Chapter 1, the heart muscle depends upon its blood supply from the coronary arteries. The coronary arteries are tubes that originate from the aorta just above the heart, and lead to a branching of smaller arteries, arterioles (tiniest arteries), and finally capillaries that provide blood-carrying oxygen and nutrients to the heart muscle. Should blood flow through the coronary arteries be reduced or stopped, as is the case during a heart attack, serious damage to the heart muscle can occur.

During a heart attack, blood flow is terminated in a coronary artery supplying blood to a portion of the myocardium (heart muscle). Within a few minutes of the cessation of blood, the heart muscle cells in that area of the heart will die. Medically, this is referred to as myocardial infarction and literally means "death of heart muscle." The heart attack may cause a disturbance in the rhythm of the heart such as fibrillation (quivering) which reduces the pumping action of the heart, or it may damage a significant portion of the myocardium and markedly impair the pumping activity of the heart. About 30% of people will die from their first heart attack or myocardial infarction.

When a major heart attack occurs with subsequent reduced pumping of the heart, blood pressure is severely lowered, and passage of blood through all organs of the body is dramatically reduced. This is commonly called cardiogenic shock. It is a clinical syndrome brought about by inadequate blood flow, which results in insufficient transportation of oxygen to all tissues and organs. It is, oftentimes, fatal. Essentially, cardiogenic shock results when the heart doesn't pump enough blood to sustain life.

A heart attack generally occurs in one of two ways. If the cholesterol deposit is so significant that blood flow in a coronary artery or one of its branches is completely stopped, a heart attack has occurred. However, the vast majority of heart attacks occur in coronary arteries which are not completely blocked by cholesterol blockages; rather, the coronary artery is only partially or modestly narrowed. At the point of the narrowing, a blood clot develops. A blood clot is also called a thrombus. The blood clot completely plugs the artery and stops blood flow, resulting in the heart attack or myocardial infarction. That is why it is so important for a person who has been diagnosed with coronary artery disease (cholesterol deposits in the coronary arteries) to take an aspirin tablet, daily. An aspirin reduces your risk of having a heart attack by lowering the potential of a blood clot to form in a partially narrowed coronary artery. Aspirin has no impact on reducing the deposition of cholesterol into the artery wall; it is primarily a blood-thinner.

At this point in the discussion, it seems appropriate to again distinguish between coronary heart disease and coronary artery disease. The terms are commonly used interchangeably, yet strictly speaking there is a difference. Coronary artery disease is the atherosclerotic plaques (cholesterol buildup) within the inner linings of the coronary arteries. Coronary heart disease is the damage to the myocardium (heart muscle) that results from the stoppage of blood flow through a diseased coronary artery or one of its branches. The stoppage of blood flow results in a heart attack by depriving the heart muscle of the oxygen and nutrients the blood delivers. After a few minutes of blood deprivation the heart muscle will die. **For the purpose of simplicity, I will use coronary heart disease throughout the remainder of this book to refer to the cholesterol plaques (i.e., atherosclerosis) in the coronary arteries.**

Atherosclerosis

Atherosclerosis, hardening of the arteries, or the accumulation of cholesterol in the artery linings are essentially all the same. In short, atherosclerosis is the clinical term used when an individual has several such blockages to varying degrees in his/her arteries. If you have been diagnosed with atherosclerosis in the coronary arteries, you have been specifically diagnosed with coronary heart disease. Remember that in addition to the coronary arteries, other arteries in the body can develop atherosclerosis including the arteries of the neck (carotid arteries), brain (cerebrovascular arteries), and legs (iliac, femoral, and popliteal arteries).

It is estimated that over 14 million Americans have diagnosed atherosclerosis in the coronary arteries (i.e., coronary heart disease) and over 4 million have atherosclerosis in the arteries of the brain, which increases the chance of stroke. *Over 75% of all cardiovascular disease deaths are the result of atherosclerosis in either the coronary (heart) or cerebrovascular (brain) arteries.*

Due to the high prevalence of atherosclerosis in the population, it is considered an epidemic. This is highlighted by the direct and indirect cost to society that atherosclerosis carries. Approximately $100 billion is spent each year for coronary heart disease victims, and approximately $50 billion for stroke victims. Considering that most cases of heart failure are caused as the result of heart attacks leading to heart muscle damage, the total direct and indirect cost for atherosclerotic-related diseases to society is over $200 billion per year. Remember that all forms of cardiovascular disease cost society about $290 billion per year.

These types of statistics are sobering and indicate the essential need for prevention and effective treatment of atherosclerosis. An individual with coronary heart disease, or atherosclerosis in any of the other arteries of the body, needs to make sure that he or she is doing everything possible to prevent the disease from causing devastating complications or even death. That is, to take measures to stabilize the existing atherosclerosis and prevent it from progressing.

To accomplish this, the first step is to understand how atherosclerosis develops. While its prevalence has increased during modern times, it is not a new disease. There is evidence that severe atherosclerosis in the coronary arteries and in the arteries of the brain was present during ancient Egyptian times (i.e., 3000 BC). This was discovered through the examinations of Egyptian mummies. In addition, the natural history of the development of atherosclerosis indicates that it begins early in life. Autopsies of young men who died in the Korean and Vietnam wars showed that atherosclerosis is present at age 18. Interestingly, evidence of its presence in prepubescent children was reported in the Bogalusa Heart Study. Doctors conducting this medical study (observational), reported the presence of atherosclerosis in the arteries (coronary and aorta) of children who died in automobile accidents.

Atherosclerosis first appears as a fatty streak, which in appearance is a yellowish accumulation of cholesterol in the lining of the artery and does not impair blood flow. It is believed that these fatty streaks that form in children and adolescents are the precursors to the more serious blockages that form later in life. The color and composition of atherosclerotic plaques is the result of specific white blood cells, called macrophages, that absorb the cholesterol that accumulates in the inner lining of an artery. These macrophages come from the blood and penetrate the inner lining of an artery. As macrophages absorb more and more cholesterol, they become yellow and are called "foam cells." Cholesterol that accumulates in foam cells is derived specifically from what is called low-density lipoprotein (LDL) cholesterol, or "bad" cholesterol. LDL-cholesterol is that portion of the total blood cholesterol that is contained in the LDL lipoprotein package

The Role of Cholesterol (LDL and HDL)

Prior to explaining how cholesterol, particularly LDL-cholesterol causes atherosclerosis, a discussion of the normal role of cholesterol in the body is timely. Cholesterol, like other forms of fat, does have important purposes in normal body function or metabolism.

Cholesterol is required by all of us for the following reasons. **Bile is manufactured from cholesterol.** Bile is a substance that is manufactured in the liver and stored in the gall bladder, and is important for the digestion of dietary fats. When we eat a meal, and food passes from our stomach to the small intestine, a hormone is released from the duodenum (the first portion of the small intestine) into the bloodstream. This hormone, called cholecystokinin, causes the gall bladder to contract, squeezing bile into a duct (the gall bladder duct) which connects to the small intestine. The bile is squirted into the small intestine and mixes with the food in the small intestine, helping to digest it so that it can be absorbed into the body.

Another important role for cholesterol is that **it is necessary for the production of certain hormones.** Testosterone, estradiol, and cortisol are all hormones produced by the body and require cholesterol for their production.

Finally, **cholesterol is an important building block of all cells.** All cells are surrounded by a cell membrane. Every day our body is producing new cells to replace those that have died (while most cells of the body reproduce, cells of the brain, spinal cord, skeletal muscle, and heart muscle do not). In order to accomplish this the body requires a certain amount of cholesterol to manufacture new cell membranes. *Since the body has the capacity to produce the amount of cholesterol that it needs, very little, if any, is required from the diet.*

In addition to cholesterol, the other major fat in the blood stream is triglyceride. Cholesterol and triglyceride are referred to as major lipids. Like cholesterol, a certain amount of triglyceride is also necessary in order for the body to function properly. Triglycerides are used by the body to produce energy. Once transported to the cells of the body, triglycerides are broken down to form energy. Triglyceride, in other words, is a fuel (like glucose) that the body uses to carry out its normal activities.

Both triglyceride and cholesterol are chemically similar to oil while blood is primarily composed of water. We all know that oil and water do not mix. Therefore, in order to dissolve and transport these fats in the bloodstream they must be contained in packages called lipoproteins. Spherically shaped, lipoproteins are composed of an outer shell of protein (referred to as apolipoprotein) and an inner core of fat (cholesterol and triglyceride). All cholesterol and triglyceride in the blood are carried in these fat packages, or lipoproteins. Lipoproteins either deliver cholesterol and triglyceride to cells in the body or help remove excess cholesterol from cells.

There are four major lipoproteins or fat packages in the blood—chylomicrons, VLDL, LDL and HDL. Low density lipoprotein (LDL) and high density lipoprotein (HDL) carry over 90% of the total cholesterol in blood. Chylomicrons and very low density lipoproteins (VLDL) carry virtually all of the triglycerides in the bloodstream. VLDL carries about 10% of the total cholesterol in blood *(Figure 8)*.

LDL contains the "bad" cholesterol because it is the lipoprotein that delivers cholesterol to the cells and is capable of delivering too much if the LDL is in high concentrations. HDL contains the "good" cholesterol because it is the lipoprotein

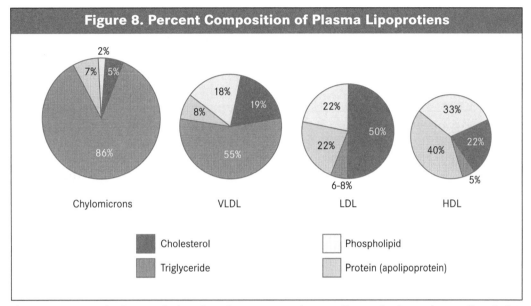

Figure 8. Percent Composition of Plasma Lipoprotiens

Chylomicrons: 2%, 7%, 5%, 86%

VLDL: 18%, 8%, 19%, 55%

LDL: 22%, 22%, 50%, 6-8%

HDL: 33%, 22%, 40%, 5%

Legend:
- Cholesterol
- Triglyceride
- Phospholipid
- Protein (apolipoprotein)

that removes cholesterol that has been stored in cells, including the cells of the coronary artery walls. HDLs prevent the accumulation of cholesterol, and HDL are actually "scavenger" lipoproteins necessary for removing cholesterol from the inner linings of arteries *(Figure 9)*.

Cholesterol is delivered to cells by LDL. Every cell has specific receptors or doors that allow LDL to enter. Upon entering the cell, the cholesterol in LDL is either used up or stored. In the case of the liver, the cholesterol can be used to manufacture bile. In the adrenal glands, testes, and ovaries, the cholesterol can be used to manufacture hormones. In most cells, the cholesterol can be used as a building block for new cell membrane development. If the cholesterol is not used, it is stored within the cell for use at a later time.

Because LDL is the lipoprotein package that delivers cholesterol to cells and, when in high concentrations, is capable of delivering too much cholesterol, it is commonly referred to

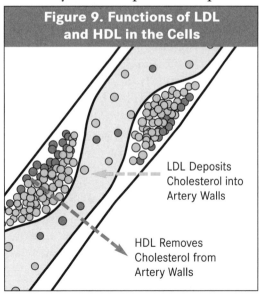

Figure 9. Functions of LDL and HDL in the Cells

LDL Deposits Cholesterol into Artery Walls

HDL Removes Cholesterol from Artery Walls

as "bad" cholesterol. Excessive amounts of cholesterol entering the inner lining of a coronary artery will be stored and eventually accumulate. As more and more accumulates, the cells in the lining of the artery become larger and begin to expand into the inner opening (lumen) of the artery. This process constitutes the beginning stages of atherosclerosis (i.e., fatty streak formation).

The cholesterol that is contained in HDL particles is referred to as "good" cholesterol because it is the cholesterol that has been removed from storage deposits in cells, including the cells of the coronary artery walls. In effect, HDLs act as scavengers to remove cholesterol from cells and prevent it from accumulating to excessive levels. HDL particles do this by binding to these cells, causing them to release stored cholesterol. When HDL-cholesterol is high in the bloodstream, this indicates that cholesterol is being effectively removed from cells. When the HDL-cholesterol is low, this indicates impaired cholesterol removal and the tendency for cholesterol to accumulate.

From this discussion, it is obvious to prefer that your LDL-cholesterol be low (generally less than 100 milligrams per deciliter, mg/dL) and your HDL-cholesterol be high (greater than 40 mg/dL). You should also be able to understand that your total cholesterol concentration is of limited value in assessing whether you are at heightened risk of developing coronary heart disease. There are individuals who have a high total cholesterol that is predominately due to a high HDL-cholesterol level. This situation is favorable since cholesterol is not likely to be accumulating in the linings of arteries. As you should be able to gather, this type of high total cholesterol does not suggest that these individuals are prone to atherosclerosis or are at an increased risk of developing coronary heart disease. Rather, it indicates just the opposite.

Conversely, there are individuals who may have a favorable total cholesterol (i.e., less than 200 mg/dL) and are at heightened risk of atherosclerosis in the coronary arteries. This is because the HDL-cholesterol is low (e.g., less than 35 mg/dL), and low HDL-cholesterol indicates that cholesterol is not being removed from the lining of arteries, increasing the likelihood of accumulation. Therefore, to assess the risk of coronary heart disease, or any form of atherosclerosis, you need to know the LDL-cholesterol number and the HDL-cholesterol number. The total cholesterol number is of limited value.

In addition to the LDL-cholesterol and HDL-cholesterol levels, the fasting blood triglyceride level is also important when assessing the lipid (or fat) profile and its association with the risk of coronary heart disease. After twelve hours of having no food or fluids other than water, your triglycerides are considered in the fasting state. In this condition, when they are greater than 200 mg/dL, they enhance the ability of LDL to deliver and deposit its cholesterol into the cell of an artery wall, and they impair the ability of HDL to remove excess cholesterol. Basically, a high triglyceride level (greater than 200 mg/dL) will shrink the size of the LDL packages, allowing them to more easily leave the blood and penetrate into the cells making up the inner lining of the arteries. Conversely, with high triglycerides, the size of the HDL packages increase, and this prevents them from effectively removing cholesterol from cells of the artery wall.

Therefore, when the lipid profile is discussed, the blood levels of LDL-cholesterol, HDL-cholesterol, and triglycerides should be taken into account. This is sometimes referred to in medical terms as the "lipid triad."

More About LDL—the "Bad" Cholesterol

Having discussed the roles of LDL, HDL, cholesterol and triglyceride, it is now the time to describe how LDL causes the development of atherosclerosis. It is interesting to understand how, and by what mechanism these "bad" cholesterol packages promote this disease. As pointed out earlier, LDL delivers cholesterol to all cells in the body. The LDL exits the blood and penetrates into the lining of the coronary artery. During this transfer some of the LDL becomes "oxidized" (i.e., oxygen molecules are added), which modifies the function of LDL. Instead of just depositing its cholesterol into the coronary artery lining, the modified or oxidized LDL initiates an inflammatory reaction. Inflammation is the body's response to injury, and the accumulation of cholesterol from LDL, particularly oxidized LDL, in the lining of a coronary artery, is injurious. Inflammation is initiated by white blood cells. The accumulating oxidized LDL attracts white blood cells from the blood to enter into the inner lining of the coronary artery. These white blood cells (called monocytes and T-lymphocytes) begin the inflammatory reaction in an attempt to reduce the injurious insult (i.e., remove oxidized LDL) and prevent it from spreading. The monocytes are referred to as macrophages when they become embedded in the lining of a coronary artery, and they act as scavengers by consuming the oxidized LDL. The macrophages also secrete chemical substances that attract more white blood cells (i.e., monocytes and T-lymphocytes) from the blood into the lining of the coronary artery. These chemical substances also cause redness and mild swelling within the inner linings of the artery (inflammation). Furthermore, when the inflammation occurs, smooth muscle cells move from the outer lining of the artery and into the inner lining. These smooth muscle cells also help to consume some of the accumulating oxidized LDL.

These processes begin to add bulk and substance to the developing atherosclerotic plaque. Actually, in the initial stages, the majority of the bulk is within the coronary artery lining and does not significantly encroach into the open space (lumen) of the coronary artery. When macrophages have taken up too much oxidized LDL, they die and become foam cells which are permanent fixtures of the atherosclerotic blockages. The smooth muscle cells that have accumulated oxidized LDL begin to secrete collagen and elastin. These are connective tissue proteins that form a scar over the accumulating cholesterol and isolate the cholesterol and inflammation from the blood and prevent the inflammation from spreading throughout the entire length of the artery. This scar also adds even more bulk to the growing obstruction. As this process continues over years the blockage, or atherosclerotic plaque, begins to invade the artery lumen (inner opening) and reduces blood flow. Of course, if the HDL blood concentration is high enough, these lipoproteins can remove some of the cholesterol that has been delivered by the LDL to the coronary artery lining and prevent it from building up and setting off this cascade of events that lead to the atherosclerotic plaque.

Many atherosclerotic plaques contain some degree of inflammation, which is very serious because inflammation makes these blockages susceptible to causing a heart attack. Generally, the inflammation predominates in the cholesterol blockages that obstruct the lumen of the coronary artery by only 30% to 50%. As pointed out previously, white blood cells, called macrophages and T-lymphocytes, manufacture and release biological chemicals (called cytokines) into the blockage site causing the inflammation and this makes the plaque very fragile. The fragility or delicacy is caused by these chemicals "breaking down" or disintegrating the scar cap over the cholesterol plaque. The thinning scar is susceptible to easily breaking open. Should a fragile blockage break apart, platelets (clotting factors) in the blood rapidly collect at the site and form a clot, or thrombus, which plugs the artery and stops blood flow. Remember, this is a heart attack if it occurs in a coronary artery or a stroke if it occurs in a brain artery.

The above paragraph introduces surprising information. It indicates that the most critical cholesterol plaques are those that occupy the inner opening (lumen) of a coronary artery by less than 50%. Of course this opposes the traditionally held belief that the larger the plaque the more likely it is to cause a heart attack. This is not true. Small plaques are more dangerous because they are inflamed and this causes them to be fragile and therefore susceptible to breaking open. *(Figure 10)*

The smaller cholesterol plaques are also dangerous because a person will not know they are present. These plaques usually do not cause angina or other symptoms. By and large, cholesterol plaque can occupy up to 70% of the lumen of a coronary artery before an individual will notice that there is a problem. Remember that what a person may notice in this case is one of the symptoms of coronary heart disease such as chest pressure or discomfort, shortness of breath, or fatigue. The reason that these symptoms are usually not present when a plaque

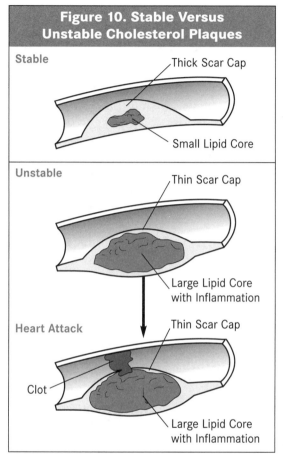

Figure 10. Stable Versus Unstable Cholesterol Plaques

Stable

Thick Scar Cap

Small Lipid Core

Unstable

Thin Scar Cap

Large Lipid Core with Inflammation

Heart Attack

Thin Scar Cap

Clot

Large Lipid Core with Inflammation

is less than 70% is because coronary arteries are able to autoregulate, depending upon the blood flow needs of the heart. Autoregulation is a process by which a coronary artery relaxes (opens up), allowing for more blood flow, or constricts (closes), decreasing blood flow. If the heart muscle has certain demands for blood, based on its degree of workload, the coronary arteries will dilate or constrict (open up or close down) to meet the blood demands. It can do this effectively, even if an atherosclerotic plaque blocks the coronary artery by up to 70%. Therefore, autoregulation can prevent one from experiencing symptoms of reduced coronary blood flow unless a plaque exceeds 70%.

As a plaque obstructs the coronary artery more than 70%, such as 80-90% or more, the artery cannot relax enough to allow for more blood flow to compensate for the blockage. Therefore, the heart muscle does not receive the blood that it requires to function properly. When this occurs, the person will usually experience chest pain or discomfort, or even shortness of breath.

This phenomenon is quite analogous to a person who has not been training and decides to run a mile. We all know that if we are not in good shape, when we attempt to run, soon the muscles in our legs begin to cramp and hurt. The reason is because the arteries of the leg feeding the muscles are not able to deliver enough blood-carrying oxygen and nutrients to satisfy the demands of the active muscle. There is also a buildup of carbon dioxide and waste products in the muscle. We experience this as muscle cramping. Since the heart is a muscle, if its demands for oxygen and nutrients and removal of waste products are not met, it will begin to cramp and hurt, and we experience this as chest pain, commonly called "angina."

Cholesterol plaques that cause angina are generally obstructing the coronary artery lumen by more than 70%, and usually have a thick scar cap surrounding the cholesterol accumulation. They tend to be older cholesterol blockages than those that obstruct the coronary artery by less than 50%. Being older, they have become sturdy and durable. This is because they are comprised of more scar tissue covering the cholesterol and inflammation than younger plaques. Also, lesser degrees of inflammation occur in these plaques allowing for a thick scar cap surrounding the cholesterol deposit. Being durable, they do not break and do not result in heart attacks. Yes, they cause the symptoms of coronary heart disease (e.g., angina, fatigue, shortness of breath), but no, they do not usually result in the catastrophic events of heart attack or death.

This prior discussion emphasizes the need for a new paradigm concerning coronary heart disease. That is, the type of atherosclerosis that causes symptoms is relatively safe, whereas the type that is free of symptoms (asymptomatic) is dangerous. However, many individuals with symptomatic atherosclerosis also will have cholesterol plaques that are not contributing to their symptoms, and these are the plaques that cause a heart attack.

Stroke

Atherosclerotic blockages in the coronary arteries, primarily small delicate ones, can lead to a heart attack. Now, you may ask, what does this have to do with stroke? The answer is very simple—most stroke results from the formation of atherosclerotic plaques in the arteries of the brain.

As in the case of a heart attack, blood is shut off to a portion of the brain because of cholesterol plaques that either completely or partially block a brain artery. A cholesterol deposit that partially blocks a brain artery may break open and prompt a blood clot to form that completely shuts off blood flow in much the same fashion as can occur in a coronary artery. This is referred to as a stroke or brain infarct. Those portions of the brain that received its blood supply from the blocked artery will die. This can be a devastating situation. It can paralyze a person or take away their strength, memory or ability to speak. Strokes resulting from atherosclerosis are referred to as ischemic strokes. Ischemia is the medical term for deficient flow of blood to a particular organ. Another type of ischemic stroke is called embolic stroke. This occurs when a blood clot forms within the heart, or on the wall of some artery in the body, and then breaks off and travels to the brain and lodges in a brain artery. It will plug the artery and shut off the flow of blood. Remember from earlier in this chapter that people who have a serious mitral valve prolapse causing significant surging backflow of blood into the left atrium have a tendency to form blood clots inside the heart chamber. These clots can travel from the heart and into the brain arteries and cause an embolic stroke. If a person survives any type of stroke, their resulting disabilities are determined by the location or portion of the brain that was deprived of blood.

There are two general types of stroke—the ischemic stroke mentioned above, (i.e., atherosclerotic or embolic) and hemorrhagic stroke. Generally, 80% of all strokes are of the ischemic variety and caused primarily by atherosclerosis, whereas 20% are hemorrhagic strokes. A hemorrhagic stroke is caused by a rupture (tear) in the wall of a brain artery, causing blood to gush or flow out into the brain tissue causing damage to the brain cells. The most common cause of hemorrhagic stroke is high blood pressure. High blood pressure can weaken the wall of a brain artery, causing it to rupture. While the consequences of both types of stroke are the same and devastating, the mechanisms are different. A hemorrhagic stroke occurs when an artery of the brain bursts. An ischemic stroke is caused by a brain artery being blocked by an atherosclerotic blockage, blood clot (thrombus) or embolus.

Sometimes hemorrhagic strokes can occur in a person who is anticoagulated. Anticoagulation means reduction in the clotting ability of the blood. There are specific drugs that are used to reduce the coagulability of blood. The most common is aspirin. However, the risk of having a hemorrhagic stroke from taking aspirin is insignificant. Generally, in a person who has a congenital defect resulting in reduced blood clotting ability, such as a hemophiliac, the risk of hemorrhagic stroke increases because microscopic blood vessels are not able to clot. Although the very smallest blood vessels (arterioles and capillaries) rupture normally, the body's normal clotting mechanism plugs the opening, preventing significant blood loss. In a hemophiliac, this does not occur effectively, and so even the smallest, tiniest rupture leads to bleeding.

Conclusion

To briefly review, there are three general types of cardiovascular diseases or defects—mechanical, electrical, and plumbing. Mechanical defects are related to either the faulty performance of the heart muscle (its contractions and relaxations) or the heart valves (their opening and closing). Electrical defects cause irregularities in the heartbeat, which disable the heart muscle's ability to properly pump blood into the body or lungs. Plumbing defects occur in the blood vessels, usually the arteries. Plumbing defects arise when the arteries become blocked to varying degrees by the buildup of cholesterol in their inner wall. This book is focused on this last category, which is the most common form of cardiovascular disease.

B

Treatment of Coronary Heart Disease and Common Misconceptions

---

Inside Section B:

Chapter 3
Diagnosing Coronary Heart Disease

While no one of any age, gender, race, religion or lifestyle is immune from coronary heart disease, the typical person who is diagnosed with it is a 50- to 60-year-old man, or a 65- to 75-year-old woman, with troublesome or frightening chest discomfort. Usually described as heaviness, pressure, squeezing, smothering or choking, this discomfort is rarely overt pain. When asked by a doctor to point out where the sensation occurs, people usually press on their chest, sometimes with clenched fists, to indicate a squeezing pain. The pain usually lasts for one to five minutes and sometimes can spread to the left shoulder, both arms, the back, neck, jaw, or teeth.

Angina

This chest discomfort or sensation is referred to medically as angina pectoris or angina and is typically induced by common physical activities such as exercise, sexual activity, or hurrying around, and common emotions such as stress, anger, or frustration. Sometimes, however, angina can be prompted by something as routine as eating a heavy meal or exposure to cold temperatures. While rest often relieves angina symptoms, sometimes angina can occur while resting. This is referred to as unstable angina. Although coronary heart disease leads to reduced blood flow through the coronary arteries (referred to as ischemia) and causes angina, some people with the disease may not experience this symptom. This type of coronary heart disease is called "silent" ischemia. Silent ischemia is dangerous because a person has no way of knowing that they have the disease and it could lead to a "silent" heart attack.

If you experience daily to weekly episodes of angina, or angina-like symptoms, you should consult with a physician. After your doctor has heard you describe the nature of the pain or discomfort, he or she will begin an investigative process to determine if coronary heart disease is present. Generally this is accomplished by getting your medical history, your family's history of heart disease, and conducting physical and laboratory examinations.

Patient History and the Physical Examination

Patient and Family Histories

The doctor will question you to determine if there is a positive family history of heart attack or stroke. Focusing on each parent, the doctor will ask you questions about the existence and extent of any heart disease and what medications were prescribed. Then the doctor will ask about each of your siblings and aunts and uncles until a complete maternal and paternal family history has been established. The doctor will also review your past medical history (prior illnesses and disorders and any previous surgical procedures).

Physical Examination

The physical examination oftentimes produces normal results, meaning that the strengths of your pulse and heartbeat are normal. When the doctor listens to your heart with a stethoscope, he or she may oftentimes hear heart sounds that are normal even if coronary heart disease is present. The doctor will also evaluate you for high blood pressure, diabetes mellitus, high blood cholesterol, smoking status and other coronary heart disease risk factors such as excess weight, a sedentary lifestyle or a type A personality. Since coronary heart disease is not readily detected through the physical exam, laboratory testing is a natural and important step in the diagnosis.

Laboratory Examination

Laboratory tests for detecting coronary heart disease fall into two categories:

- noninvasive
- invasive

Noninvasive Testing

Noninvasive tests are usually done first and are generally given by specially trained technicians or nurses. They can be performed in the doctor's office. The results of these tests are interpreted by physicians. Noninvasive tests useful for diagnosing coronary heart disease include:

- electrocardiogram (EKG or ECG)
- ambulatory electrocardiography (Holter monitoring)
- exercise stress test
- echocardiography (with or without exercise)
- Doppler ultrasonography

► thallium scanning (with or without exercise)
► magnetic resonance imaging (MRI)
► electron-beam tomography
► radionuclide ventriculography
► position emission tomography (PET) scanning

While we will not discuss each of these noninvasive testing procedures, a review of the most commonly used will be briefly summarized. They include the EKG, stress test and radionuclide (i.e., thallium or pyrophosphate technetium 99m) scanning.

EKG

The electrocardiogram (EKG) is usually the first test to be performed. The electrocardiogram examines the electrical events within your heart that may indicate coronary heart disease. It records the electrical activity during a one-to-two-minute period. By showing any electrical deviation consistent with abnormal contracting and relaxing of the heart muscle, the EKG may detect coronary heart disease in about 50% of patients who truly have the disease. Another way of explaining this is that 50% of people with coronary heart disease have completely normal EKG results.

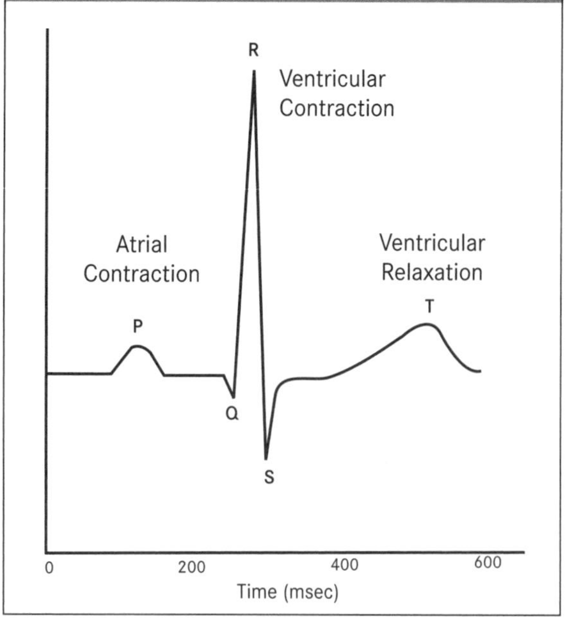

The typical electrocardiogram (Figure 11) has three components per heartbeat:

► P-wave (atrial contraction)
► QRS complex (ventricular contraction)
► T-wave (ventricular relaxation)

The P-wave represents contraction of the atria (reservoirs) of the heart. The P-wave signals when the atria contract and deposit blood into the ventricles.

The second part of the electro-cardiogram is the QRS complex. This represents the synchronized contraction of the right ventricle as it ejects blood into the pulmonary artery and the left ventricle as it

Figure 11. The Electrocardiogram Examines the Electrical Activity Within the Heart

ejects blood into the aorta. Blood that is ejected from the right ventricle into the pulmonary artery enters into the lungs where it is oxygenated. The blood that is ejected from the left ventricle into the aorta carries oxygenated blood to all other tissues and organs in the body.

The final component of the EKG is the T-wave. The T-wave represents the relaxation, or "recovery" of the left and right ventricles.

In addition to assisting the doctor in discovering the presence of coronary heart disease, the electrocardiogram is useful for detecting arrhythmias or rhythm disturbances of the heart.

Another type of EKG testing is referred to as the "continuous EKG." This EKG records the electrical activity of the heart over a 12 to 24 hour period. A portable EKG machine is attached to and carried by the person being tested. The machine is called a Holter monitor and allows for evaluating the heart's electrical activity over long periods of time. It is generally used primarily for detecting rhythm disturbances rather than coronary heart disease.

Stress Test

Another regularly used laboratory test for the diagnosis of coronary heart disease is the exercise stress test. This is simply an EKG performed during and after exercise on a treadmill or a stationary cycle. The EKG electrodes are attached to a person's arms, legs, and chest, and he/she will begin walking on a treadmill. Gradually the speed and the incline will be increased until the person is running in place on an incline. Exercise is better than rest for allowing an EKG to reveal coronary heart disease since it becomes most evident after exercising. Generally, the exercise that a person who has coronary heart disease performs will cause ST segment depression of the EKG that may not have been observed on the resting EKG. An ST segment depression is an abnormal electrical change in the impulse of the heart that usually signifies the presence of coronary heart disease. During the stress test, the speed or resistance of the equipment (e.g., treadmill) is increased while the person's blood pressure and potential angina symptoms are monitored. Chest discomfort, shortness of breath, premature fatigue or dizziness usually assists in determining the pressure and severity of the coronary heart disease. While the stress test laboratory procedure is far more accurate at identifying coronary heart disease than a resting EKG, it does carry false negative results. A false negative result means that the test revealed no presence of the disease, even though the disease is present. A false negative stress test may be due to small arteries called "collaterals" that develop in the myocardium to compensate for large blockages in the coronary arteries. For unknown reasons, a false negative result occurs more frequently in women. Conversely, some people who do not have coronary heart disease may have a false positive stress test—a test that indicates the disease is present, even though it is not. A false positive stress test may occur in people with rapid heart rates (tachycardia), or women at the time of menopause, or people taking certain types of heart medication (digitalis).

The exercise stress test is usually done in a doctor's office and lasts about 15 to 30 minutes.

Radionuclide Testing

Radionuclide scanning or testing is a noninvasive test for helping to diagnose coronary heart disease with much more sensitivity than the resting EKG or exercise stress test. It allows the doctor to visualize the heart and coronary arteries. It is oftentimes used to evaluate the condition of the heart after a heart attack and therefore, the presence of coronary heart disease. It is normally performed in a hospital or clinic and lasts from approximately 30 minutes to two hours. A radioactive substance (either thallium or pyrophosphate technetium 99) is injected into a vein (in the arm or leg), and a scanning camera takes a series of pictures of the heart.

The radioactive substance collects in the heart muscle that is normal with a good blood supply. It will not collect in areas of the heart that are damaged (because of a heart attack) or do not receive adequate blood supply. By reviewing the pictures, the doctor can identify areas of the heart that do not receive sufficient blood because of narrowed coronary arteries, or are scarred because of a prior heart attack. The procedure is safe and the amount of radioactivity that a person undergoing this procedure is exposed to is equal to that amount associated with a chest x-ray. A radionuclide scan can also be done in conjunction with exercise.

Invasive Testing

The other major category of laboratory testing to aid in the diagnosis of coronary heart disease is *invasive* testing. These tests are performed when the results of noninvasive testing are inconclusive or the doctor requires more information about the extent and location of the coronary artery blockages. They are also done when heart bypass surgery, angioplasty, or other open heart surgery is being seriously considered. Invasive testing for diagnosing coronary heart disease is coronary angiography and requires catheterization of the coronary arteries.

Coronary Catheterization

Coronary catheterization is the invasive procedure that allows doctors to perform angiography, or visualization of blood flowing through the coronary arteries. This procedure is the gold standard for assessing cholesterol blockages (plaques) in the coronary arteries. This is the so-called heart (or cardiac) catheterization and it provides the doctor with a visual picture of the insides of the coronary arteries. With this testing procedure, the doctor can actually see the presence and extent of cholesterol plaques.

The risks of coronary catheterization are very low. They are usually outweighed by the benefit of knowing the exact condition of your heart and if blockages exist in the coronary arteries. If you are scheduled for this procedure, your doctor will most likely discuss any potential risks and side effects in advance, and you will be asked to sign a legal consent form. Side effects are very rare and occur in less than 2% of patients undergoing the procedure. Possible risks that can occur as a result of coronary catheterization include excessive bleeding or blood clot formation, perforation of the heart muscle or coronary artery, abnormal heartbeats, allergic reactions to the x-ray-sensitive liquid, and although extremely rare, a heart attack or stroke.

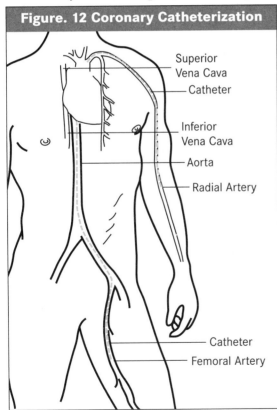

Figure. 12 Coronary Catheterization

Superior Vena Cava

Catheter

Inferior Vena Cava

Aorta

Radial Artery

Catheter

Femoral Artery

The procedure is performed in a catheterization laboratory at a hospital. In the catheterization laboratory, a patient is draped with sterile sheets and only the patch of skin where the catheter or tube will be inserted is exposed. The doctor, as well as nurses and technicians, wear sterile gowns, gloves, and masks. The patient is awake, although relaxed (a sedative is given) during the procedure.

Once underway, the procedure itself takes an hour or less. The area of skin where the catheter or tube will be inserted is numbed with a local anesthetic so no pain is felt. Normally this will be a patch of skin above the femoral artery, which is located in the groin area. Sometimes the doctor may choose to insert the catheter in the radial artery, located in the lower forearm or elbow region (*Figure 12*). In this case, the skin above the radial artery will be numbed with a local anesthetic. The patient will most likely remain awake during the entire procedure because it may be necessary for him/her to hold his/her breath, move his/her body slightly, or cooperate in some other similar way.

An introducing tube, called a sheath, is inserted directly into the artery (i.e., femoral artery or radial artery) and it is through this tube that another tube or catheter (called a diagnostic catheter) is inserted. The diagnostic catheter is gently moved from the femoral or radial artery into the aorta and inserted into one of the two coronary ostia (openings) which give rise to the right and left coronary arteries of the heart. Sometimes patients feel a small amount of pressure, usually in the chest, but the sensation usually passes quickly and generally no further pain or discomfort is felt.

Cholesterol blockages in the coronary arteries (i.e., coronary artery disease) are identified by inserting the tip of the diagnostic catheter into the opening of the coronary artery (or ostium) at the site of the aorta and injecting an x-ray contrast fluid *(Figure 13)*. While this contrast fluid is being injected into the coronary artery, some people experience a hot flash, which usually subsides within a few

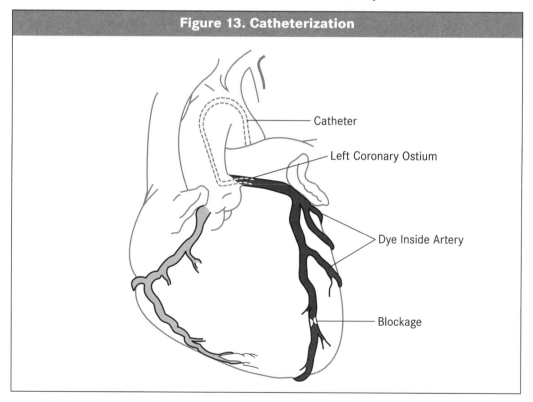

Figure 13. Catheterization

Catheter

Left Coronary Ostium

Dye Inside Artery

Blockage

seconds. An x-ray monitor will show the inside of the artery and readily reveal any existing blockages. During this stage of the procedure the x-ray equipment may be rotated at various angles around the body so that the doctor can visualize, three-dimensionally, the extent of any cholesterol blockages that may exist throughout the coronary artery *(Figure 14 and Figure 15)*.

When the cardiac catheterization procedure is completed, the doctor removes the diagnostic catheter and introducing sheath from the femoral or radial artery. If the catheter was inserted in the radial artery of the arm, the doctor stitches the artery, then closes the skin and inserts additional stitches. If the catheter was inserted in the groin into the femoral artery through a needle, they are removed and a nurse will clamp or press down firmly on the insertion area for about 15 to 20 minutes to stop any bleeding. Sometimes a sandbag or pressure bandage is placed on the insertion site before the patient returns to the recovery room.

Generally, after the catheterization procedure, a person will not have any pain. Usually in less than an hour, the doctor will provide the patient with specific information such as the presence or extent of the coronary heart disease. The

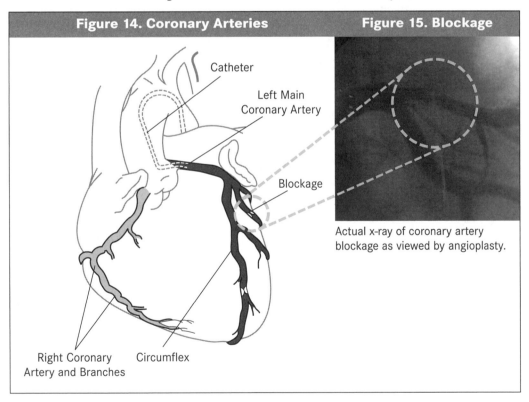

Figure 14. Coronary Arteries

Figure 15. Blockage

Catheter

Left Main Coronary Artery

Blockage

Right Coronary Artery and Branches

Circumflex

Actual x-ray of coronary artery blockage as viewed by angioplasty.

patient must remain lying down in the recovery room for about four to six hours and then, most likely, will be able to go home the same day. Only a small number of people spend the night in the hospital. A small bruise or an almond-size lump may be noticed under the skin at the insertion site over the groin. The skin in that area will usually be black and blue. These are common side effects after a cardiac catheterization and usually disappear within a few weeks.

For the first few days following this invasive procedure, heavy lifting and strenuous exercise activity should be avoided. After that brief period, most people are able to return to their regular daily activities.

The cardiac catheterization procedure is important for diagnosing the presence of cholesterol blockages in the coronary arteries, and other potential heart problems. However, it can also be used for the treatment of coronary heart disease by a procedure called balloon angioplasty (percutaneous transmural coronary angioplasty, PTCA—this treatment is explained in detail in Chapter 5).

Briefly, angioplasty, or PTCA, is a procedure to open up, or dilate, partially blocked coronary arteries, and is done during the cardiac catheterization procedure. The physician inserts a guiding catheter, or tube, through the introducing sheath that is inserted in the femoral artery to the opening of the coronary artery (ostium) to be dilated. Another smaller catheter, which retains an uninflated balloon on its tip, is inserted into the guiding catheter. This balloon catheter is inserted and positioned at the location in the coronary artery that is obstructed. An x-ray contrasting fluid is then injected into the coronary artery from the tip of this catheter. An x-ray monitor is used to visualize the coronary artery and takes pictures of the coronary arteries. Once the balloon is positioned at the most narrowed, or blocked, portion of the coronary artery, it is inflated. The doctor may inflate and deflate the balloon several times to "open-up," or dilate, the coronary artery blockage.

Sometimes the balloon may not keep the blocked artery open and a stent may be used. A stent resembles a spring and is placed over the tip of a balloon catheter. When the balloon is inflated at the blockage site, the stent expands and is partially imbedded in the artery wall, allowing it to remain open. The balloon is then deflated and the balloon catheter is removed.

Emergency Room Procedure

Obviously, the ultimate indicator of coronary heart disease is a myocardial infarction or heart attack. Often, the patient was engaged in some form of vigorous physical exercise, recovering from a medical or surgical illness, or was under extreme emotional stress immediately or within a couple of hours prior to the heart attack.

A heart attack can occur any time of the day or night, but occurs more frequently during the predawn hours or a few hours before awakening. During a heart attack a patient is oftentimes weak, profusely sweating, nauseated, and quite anxious. Severe chest pain is the most common signal of a heart attack. Sometimes the pain is so severe that a patient may describe it as the worst pain they have ever felt. The pain is generally heavy, squeezing, or crushing, although sometimes it will be described as stabbing or burning. It is similar to the pain of angina, although it is usually more severe and lasts longer. Generally in the central portion of the chest, the pain occasionally radiates to the arms. Because of this location, heart attacks and indigestion are sometimes mistaken for one another. If you have been diagnosed with coronary heart disease and you experience chest pain or discomfort, always assume it is cardiac pain and not indigestion.

A heart attack can occur in three ways:
▶ when the blood flowing through a coronary artery is completely stopped because of a cholesterol blockage,
▶ when a blood clot has formed and lodged in the coronary artery and stopped blood flow,
▶ or a combination of both (this is the most common way a heart attack occurs).

Blood clots are likely to form in the areas of the coronary artery where there are cholesterol blockages (plaques). When blood flow is stopped in a coronary artery, all of the heart cells that rely on the oxygen and nutrients carried by the blood—from the point of the blockage downstream—are in jeopardy of dying *(Figure 16)*. When heart muscle cells die, their contents slowly accumulate in the blood. Certain proteins are contained in the heart muscle cells and when they are detected in the bloodstream, it is indicative of a heart attack. These proteins are called cardiac markers and include creatinine kinase—MB (CK-MB), myoglobin, and troponins T and I.

When a person is taken to the emergency room for a suspected heart attack,

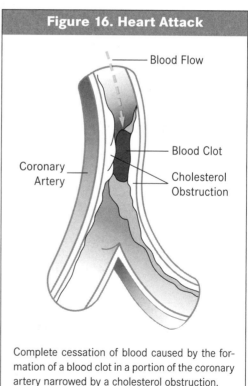

Figure 16. Heart Attack

Blood Flow

Blood Clot

Coronary Artery

Cholesterol Obstruction

Complete cessation of blood caused by the formation of a blood clot in a portion of the coronary artery narrowed by a cholesterol obstruction.

the emergency room doctor makes the diagnosis based on an EKG, the history of the chest discomfort and the blood concentrations of these "cardiac markers." If a person is having, or has had a heart attack within the past several hours, these proteins will usually be present in the bloodstream.

It sometimes takes several hours for a patient in the emergency room to be appropriately evaluated for the possibility of having had a heart attack. The patient's spouse, relatives, or friends are oftentimes anxious during this period, yet no more so than the emergency room staff who are attempting to make an accurate diagnosis of a heart attack, or not. The time delay for the diagnosis may mean that the EKG changes were not conclusive and/or the levels of the cardiac markers did not reach the peak concentration in the blood necessary to make an accurate diagnosis. It may take time for the body to demonstrate the signs (i.e., EKG changes, serum cardiac markers) that a heart attack occurred. No one wants to make a wrong diagnosis. The wrong treatment for a heart attack could cause other major medical problems. Therefore, the patience and understanding by the potential heart attack victim's relatives and spouse are appreciated by all emergency room staff.

Cardiac catheterization can also be used in emergency situations of heart attack. When a doctor in the emergency room feels that a heart attack (myocardial infarction) is occurring, he may rush the patient to the cardiac catheterization lab. The cardiologist will insert a balloon catheter through the groin or arm, into the coronary artery, and inflate the balloon to open up the artery. If used at the appropriate time, the completely blocked coronary artery is opened with resumption of blood flow and the salvaging of the "at risk" myocardium.

Thrombolytic therapy that dissolves blood clots, or thrombi, that are blocking the flow of blood through the narrowed coronary artery may also be administered during a heart attack. These clot-busting medicines include streptokinase, urokinase and tissue plasminogen activator (t-PA). They are usually given in the emergency room by being injected into a vein in the arm. If this is done within a relatively short period after the onset of the heart attack, the blood clot is dissolved and blood flow is resumed. Damage to the heart muscle is minimized. These blood clot dissolvers are sometimes called lytic agents because they lyse (break-up) the blood clot. Complications may occur in a small percentage of patients receiving thrombolytic therapy. These include fever, excessive bleeding at the injection site (i.e., vein) or internal bleeding.

Conclusion

Coronary heart disease can be very deceptive. It can exist for years before it is detected and once it has been discovered, it may be too late. A heart attack oftentimes is the first indication of coronary heart disease. Approximately 30% of people will die following a heart attack. For the survivors—the coronary heart disease and its complications can be treated. The first step of course is through accurate diagnosis. Self-diagnosis of this disease begins by monitoring your body's reaction to such everyday activities as physical exercise and emotional changes (e.g., stress). Chest pain, shortness of breath, dizziness, and fatigue that persist for a long period of time are your first indicators that a visit to the doctor is necessary. From this first visit, an accurate diagnosis may require a variety of sometimes extensive testing. **Nonetheless, the process for diagnosing and detecting this disease is not nearly as cumbersome or painful as ignoring the symptoms can be.**

Chapter 4
Common Misconceptions about
Coronary Heart Disease

Chapter 3 has provided the reader an overview of how a physician diagnoses or identifies the presence of coronary heart disease. Since this book is directed primarily at people who have been diagnosed with this disease, many of the readers will have had experience in how the medical profession treats and manages it. Chapter 5 will explain the various treatment options and their purposes. Some treatments are directed at making the patient feel better while others are for the purpose of reducing the risk of further complications, including the most devastating, **death**. However, before discussing these treatment approaches, it is necessary to bring the reader up-to-date on the most recent information and research on coronary heart disease. This latest information has dramatically changed our understanding of the disease and therefore, how it should be **effectively treated**. Unfortunately, this information has also given rise to several misconceptions.

There are six common misconceptions accepted by mainstream society and the media concerning coronary heart disease. The first one is certainly the greatest obstacle physicians must overcome in order to affect coronary heart disease's demise as the number one killer in this country. Yet, the remaining five are equally as obstructive to our country's battle against this epidemic.

Accepting this new information as factual is not easy. Doing so requires a shift in some commonly held beliefs that most Americans find very comforting. It's a lot easier to accept being diagnosed with a disease if it has a routine surgical or medical cure. For instance, if your doctor tells you that you have an inflamed gallbladder, yet all that is required is a basic surgical procedure of removal (cholecystectomy), you will be concerned, but you won't feel that your life is threatened. The same holds true for coronary heart disease. Yet, the comfort in the "cures" for coronary heart disease is based upon false notions. As Arthur Koestler [1]

---

[1] Arthur Koestler (1905-1983) British author and journalist. Author of *Darkness at Noon*. Member of the voluntary Euthanasia Society.

said "Nothing is more sad than the death of an illusion." And the following six common misconceptions, while critical to understand, may astound you.

1. Heart Bypass Surgery and Angioplasty Cure, Or Partially Cure, Coronary Heart Disease

Generally, this is false. Heart bypass surgery and angioplasty are usually performed on atherosclerotic blockages greater than 70%, so they basically alleviate the *symptoms* of coronary heart disease. These procedures increase the blood flow through the coronary arteries and can reduce chest discomfort (i.e., angina) and shortness of breath (i.e., dyspnea). If you have been diagnosed with coronary heart disease and you have experienced chest pain or discomfort, you may be recommended for angioplasty or heart bypass surgery—and rightfully so. These procedures will generally make you feel better. However, after one of these surgical procedures, even though the quality of your daily life is markedly improved (you can breathe more easily or you are free of chest pain), you are not protected from having a subsequent coronary event such as a heart attack or sudden death. In other words, these surgical procedures have little effect on prolonging life. Only in the case of heart bypass surgery when a left main coronary artery (the largest segment of the left coronary artery) blockage is bypassed or if more than three of the major coronary artery branches are bypassed, is the risk of death *modestly* reduced. Also, only if angioplasty is performed during, or immediately prior to or after a heart attack (i.e., an emergency situation), will the risk of death be modestly reduced. Most heart bypass and angioplasty procedures in this country are performed, however, on an elective basis, not an emergency situation.

The major reason these procedures have little impact on reducing the risk of further complications, including death, is that they do not treat the cholesterol plaques most likely to rupture and cause catastrophic problems. Remember from Chapter 2, that plaques that are less than 50% are the most likely locations for a heart attack to occur, and these procedures do not bypass or open-up plaques of this degree.

The evidence for these relatively disappointing outcomes from heart bypass surgery and angioplasty comes from controlled interventional clinical studies. There have been several of these types of studies conducted that evaluated the effectiveness of coronary artery bypass surgery or angioplasty on heart attack rate, death from coronary heart disease, and rate of hospitalizations required because of coronary heart disease complications. The following is a list of the most important of these studies and their results with references so that you can, should you desire, review them for your own satisfaction.

Heart Bypass Surgery Studies

Coronary Artery Surgery Study (CASS)
Demonstrated that bypass surgery reduced neither death nor heart attack in patients with stable coronary heart disease. Source: *New England Journal of Medicine*, Volume 310, pages 750-758, 1984.

Veterans Administration Cooperative Study (VACS)
Concluded that coronary artery bypass surgery did not improve overall survival of patients. Even patients with more than three blocked coronary arteries did not benefit from it. Only patients with a blockage in the main portion of the left coronary artery benefited relative to reduced mortality from bypass surgery. Source: *New England Journal of Medicine*, Volume 311, pages 1333-1340, 1984.

European Coronary Surgery Study (ECSS)
Observed that bypass surgery did not improve survival for patients with single or two-vessel coronary artery disease. Only patients with three-vessel coronary artery disease or a blockage in the left main coronary artery benefited modestly from bypass surgery. Source: *The Lancet*, Volume 2, pages 1173-1179, 1982.

Balloon Angioplasty Studies

Atorvastatin versus Revascularization Treatment (AVERT) Study
Demonstrated that aggressive lowering of "bad" cholesterol (i.e., LDL) was more effective for reducing coronary heart disease events than balloon angioplasty. Source: *New England Journal of Medicine*, Volume 341, pages 70-76, 1999.

Randomized Intervention Treatment of Angina (RITA-2) Trial
Demonstrated that patients receiving balloon angioplasty experienced more deaths and heart attacks than patients not receiving angioplasty, i.e., those who only received standard care with medications. Source: *The Lancet*; Volume 350, pages 461-468, 1997.

Angioplasty Compared to Medicine (ACME) Trial
Observed that death, heart attack, and repeat of angioplasty was 35% higher in patients receiving balloon angioplasty compared to patients not undergoing angioplasty and receiving just standard medicines. Source: *New England Journal of Medicine*, Volume 326, pages 10-16, 1992.

Angioplasty with Stents

Editorial; Alice K. Jacobs, M.D.: "To date, however, it is disappointing that no study has shown that stents favorably influence mortality." Source: *New England Journal of Medicine*, Volume 341, pages 2005-2006, 1999.

Three randomized interventional studies examining the effect of stent placement on coronary heart disease outcomes:

> Summaries: observed higher rates of death and heart attack than anticipated among patients receiving stent implantation. Sources: *New England Journal of Medicine*, Volume 331, pages 489-495, 1994; Volume 339, pages 1672-1678, 1998; Volume 341, pages 1949-1956, 1999.

2. The Severity of Atherosclerotic Coronary Blockages Is a Good Indicator of the Likelihood of a Heart Attack

Actually, the opposite is true. Clinical research studies have consistently shown that heart attacks are most often prompted by blockages of less than 50%. Clinical studies have revealed that 65% of all heart attacks occur at the site of atherosclerotic blockages that are under 50% and that 90% of all heart attacks occur at the site of atherosclerotic blockages that are less than 70%. These clinical investigations have confirmed that in the majority of people who have had heart attacks, the "culprit" blockage (the blockage causing the heart attack) was only mildly obstructing the coronary artery. Therefore, mild coronary artery disease can be very serious because it can and often leads to a heart attack. As pointed out in Chapter 2, these less obstructive blockages usually have a greater degree of inflammation associated with them than the more obstructive blockages. It is the inflammation that makes atherosclerotic blockages fragile and highly susceptive to rupture, and subsequent myocardial infarction.

I suggest that cardiologists stop referring to cholesterol blockages in the coronary arteries greater than 70% as *significant disease*. The word significant infers gravity or implies heightened risk of consequences. This is not true for coronary heart disease. Cardiologists should refer to blockages greater than 70% as "ponderous" or "bulky" since they oftentimes cause chest heaviness and shortness of breath. The blockages in the coronary arteries that are less than 50% (cardiologists generally refer to these plaques as minor coronary artery disease or coronary irregularities), should be referred to as significant or potentially serious.

3. Cardiovascular Disease Is Primarily a Man's Disease

The truth is that heart and blood vessel diseases are more prevalent in women. The notion that cardiovascular disease is a man's disease probably stems from the fact that men do suffer heart attacks an average of 10 to 15 years before women, which places them at a higher risk *earlier* in life. A woman's risk increases as menopause approaches (possibly as a result of losing the protective effect of estrogen) and continues to rise with age.

Recent studies demonstrate that most women fear breast cancer more than cardiovascular disease. How many women would still feel more threatened by breast cancer if they knew the real statistics? Remember, 1 in 26 women will die of breast cancer while 1 in 2 women will die of cardiovascular disease. Breast cancer is a serious and devastating disease but it should not overshadow the significance of cardiovascular disease. Women need to recognize the seriousness of heart and blood vessel diseases—and "stack the deck" in their favor to reduce their risk of either developing the disease or further complications if they have the disease.

4. The Only Benefit of Cholesterol-Lowering Medicines Is Reducing the Blood Cholesterol Level

Cholesterol-lowering medications called statins actually prevent heart attacks and strokes. Should you have coronary heart disease, the primary reason to take statins is because they stabilize the cholesterol plaques in your coronary arteries that are most likely to cause a heart attack. Even though, in general, blockages of less than 50% are not termed by cardiologists to be significant, you should consider them serious. When you take a statin you are giving yourself the best possible guarantee of preventing a future coronary event because these drugs stabilize the most threatening plaques. The statins convert fragile cholesterol plaques into more durable plaques.

5. Cholesterol-Lowering Medicines (Statins) Are Associated with Serious Side Effects

The facts surrounding the side-effect issue are that less than 1% of those taking these medications could *potentially* develop side effects. The actual statistics are listed in the *PDR (Physicians' Desk Reference)*. Furthermore, if a patient develops one of the adverse side effects (liver inflammation and/or muscle pain or weakness), when the medicine is stopped, the liver or muscle normalizes. Your doctor will periodically (every three to six months) monitor your blood for determining if these side effect(s) are occurring. Should the blood test indicate yes, the medicine will be stopped, or the dosage lowered, and the side effect(s) will resolve without permanent damage. *Therefore, no one should fear taking a statin because of a potential serious untoward effect.*

There are, however, certain medical conditions—existing liver disease, skeletal muscle disease and certain kidney diseases, and the use of certain drugs—erythromycin (an antibiotic), cyclosporine (an immunosuppressive), and ketoconazole (an antifungal)—that preclude a person from taking a statin. Grapefruit juice consumption can also increase the risk of a statin causing a side effect. In other words, if you are taking a statin, drink apple, pineapple, or orange juice. Your doctor is well aware of these circumstances and will not prescribe a statin if you have one of those medical conditions or are currently taking other medicines that would interact adversely with a statin. Most prescription medicines carry some side effect risk. This is one major reason that they can only be obtained through a prescription. Statins are some of the safer prescription medicines.

6. Only High Blood Cholesterol Levels Are Linked to Coronary Heart Disease and Heart Attack

There are individuals at risk for coronary heart disease who have so-called normal or low total cholesterol levels (under 200 mg/dL). As you have and will continue to discover throughout this book, high LDL-cholesterol ("bad" cholesterol) is causally related to the development of coronary heart disease, and lowering it should be your primary goal to improving your chances of not having a heart attack. In addition, there are other significant modifiable risk factors that you should strive to minimize or manage in your life. They are: high blood pressure, diabetes, smoking, low HDL-cholesterol ("good" cholesterol), and obesity. Increasing age and family history of early heart disease (a parent or sibling less than 55 years old [if male] or 65 years old [if female]), are risk factors; however, obviously they are not modifiable, and therefore, when present should make one work even harder to reduce the modifiable risk factors.

Low or normal total cholesterol blood levels should not give one the impression that their risk of coronary heart disease is low. Blood levels in the range if 170 or 180 mg/dL can be deceiving because the HDL-cholesterol is quite low (20-30 mg/dL). Therefore, ignore the level of total cholesterol. Being either high or low may not give you an accurate picture of your coronary heart disease risk. Determine and know the LDL-cholesterol, first and foremost, and secondly the HDL-cholesterol and fasting triglyceride levels.

Based on what was just presented, the over-the-counter total cholesterol testing kits, while giving you the total cholesterol number, may be of little value for some people who have either very high or very low HDL-cholesterol levels.

Conclusion

As stated at the beginning of this chapter, accepting some or all of what I have written may not be easy. We have all been inundated with information that strongly suggests that these common misconceptions are truths. However, I assure you, the facts that you have just read have all been recently identified in controlled medical studies and the results published in the leading, most well-respected medical journals. Accepting these misconceptions has helped to drive the conventional treatment of coronary heart disease. Once these issues are better understood and the misconception resolved, perhaps both the treatment and diagnosis of this destructive disease will be altered accordingly, and put us on the path toward eliminating it as the number one risk to your health and longevity.

Chapter 5
Treating Coronary Heart Disease

Now that the reader has been brought up-to-date on the most recent information about coronary heart disease and its major clinical consequence, heart attack, the various approaches to treating it and reducing the risk of its complications will be summarized.

Upon diagnosing coronary heart disease, doctors will first explain the disease to their patients and reassure them that with their cooperation, it can be treated. The treatment traditionally involves prescribing specific therapies directed at alleviating the symptoms of the disease as well as encouraging patients to adopt a lifestyle that will help them cope with the symptoms. For coronary heart disease, the symptoms that can occur, although not always, include chest discomfort, tightness, heaviness or pain (referred to as angina), shortness of breath (referred to as dyspnea) and fatigue. Usually, the symptoms are brought on by physical or emotional exertion. The physical activity that can prompt angina or dyspnea can range from something as simple as getting up from a chair, to answering the phone to climbing stairs or shoveling snow. These symptoms can also be induced by emotions ranging from worry and anxiety to full-scale anger. Sometimes these symptoms can occur after meals or exposure to cold. They may even occur at rest, which is referred to as unstable angina.

The presence of angina is different from a heart attack. As previously described in Chapter 2, angina occurs when blood flow through the coronary arteries is deficient. This happens primarily when the heart's requirement for blood is not met, as occurs when a patient is exercising or going through emotional stress. The deficient blood flow through the coronary arteries and to the heart muscle causes temporary chest discomfort (angina). The deficient blood flow is caused by one or more cholesterol plaques in the coronary arteries. A heart attack (myocardial infarction) is caused by the complete stoppage of blood flow through a coronary artery (a blood clot forms on the top of a cholesterol blockage, plugging up the artery). The lack of blood flow (and the oxygen it carries) to a portion of the heart muscle causes death of the muscle if the flow is not restored quickly. Should some of the heart muscle die, it is replaced with scar tissue which will impair the ability of the heart to pump blood *(Figure 17)*. If a substantial amount of the heart muscle dies, the heart will not be able to pump blood sufficient enough to sustain life.

At this point, it becomes essential for the reader to understand that there is a huge difference between treating symptoms of coronary heart disease and treating the underlying disease (i.e., atherosclerosis) that can result in a heart attack. A good example for illustrating this difference is using the analogy of how bronchitis is treated. Bronchitis is an infection of the bronchial tubes in the lung and results in the symptoms of coughing, congestion, fever, lethargy and breathing difficulty. A doctor can treat the symptoms by prescribing aspirin, which reduces the fever and the pain, an antihistamine, which reduces the mucous secretions and a decongestant which shrinks nasal membranes and allows you to breathe more easily. These medications will make you feel better. However, they will not cure the underlying disease or the infection of the bronchial tubes. In order to do that, an antibiotic is generally necessary. The antibiotic destroys the infective agent causing the bronchitis and the associated symptoms.

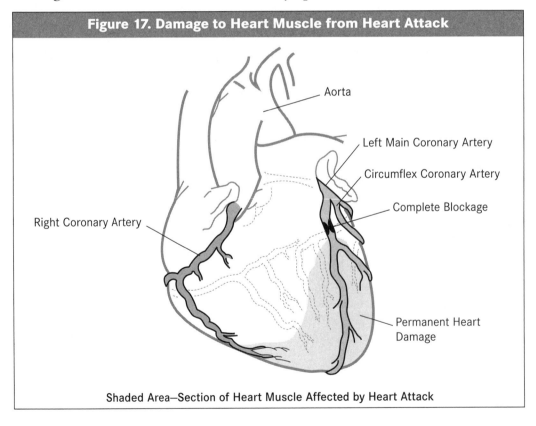

Figure 17. Damage to Heart Muscle from Heart Attack

Aorta

Left Main Coronary Artery

Circumflex Coronary Artery

Complete Blockage

Right Coronary Artery

Permanent Heart Damage

Shaded Area—Section of Heart Muscle Affected by Heart Attack

While the primary goal of treating coronary heart disease is symptomatic relief, most people believe that this approach is also treating the underlying disease (i.e., atherosclerosis). **This is not true**, and this chapter will hopefully apprise you of this distinction and make you more dedicated to accepting the therapies most effective in treating the atherosclerosis.

Treating the Symptoms

The prior example of treating the symptoms of bronchitis versus the cause of this disease (i.e., bacterial infection) is useful for describing how coronary heart disease is treated. The symptoms (e.g., angina) can be effectively treated with bypass surgery or angioplasty, and certain medications known as nitrates, beta-blockers, and calcium channel blockers. The most well-known nitrate is nitroglycerin. Nitrates are "vasodilators" or medicines that increase the size of the inner opening (lumen) of coronary arteries and allow more flow of blood. Like nitrates, calcium channel blockers are also vasodilators. They increase the opening or diameter of the artery and improve blood flow. Calcium channel blockers also effectively lower blood pressure.

Examples of calcium channel-blockers are:
- amlodipine
- nicardipine
- nifedipine
- diltiazem
- verapamil
- isradipine

Beta-blockers are a class of heart medicines useful for treating the symptoms of angina by slowing the heart beat and reducing the heart's workload. Examples of beta blockers are sotalol, timolol, propanolol, betaxolol, atenolol, metoprolol, and bisoprolol.

These classes of drugs help to relieve the symptoms of coronary heart disease although, it is important to emphasize once again, that they do not treat the underlying cause—atherosclerosis. Surgical treatments for the symptoms of coronary heart disease include angioplasty and coronary bypass surgery. **They are quite effective in alleviating the symptoms (not treating the atherosclerosis) of the disease.**

Figure 18. Mammary Artery Bypass Grafting Surgery

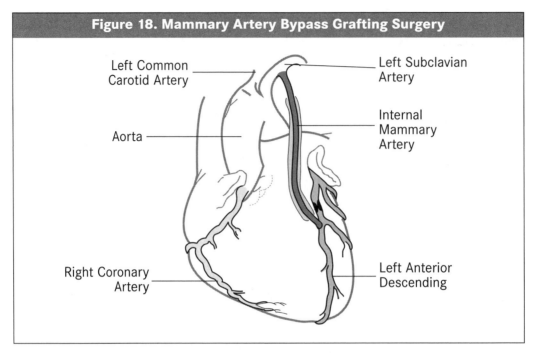

Left Common Carotid Artery

Aorta

Right Coronary Artery

Left Subclavian Artery

Internal Mammary Artery

Left Anterior Descending

Figure 19. Saphenous Vein Bypass Grafting Surgery

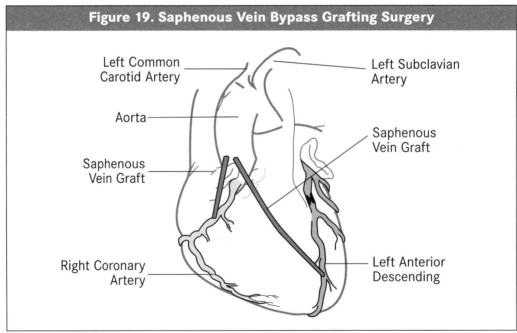

Left Common Carotid Artery

Aorta

Saphenous Vein Graft

Right Coronary Artery

Left Subclavian Artery

Saphenous Vein Graft

Left Anterior Descending

Surgical Treatments

Coronary Artery Bypass Grafting (CABG) Surgery

Coronary Artery Bypass Grafting (CABG) surgery is generally performed on patients who have multiple cholesterol deposits of 70% or more in their coronary arteries. Their angina tends to be severe enough to interfere with daily activities. Also, it is a procedure performed on patients with unstable angina (remember that this is chest discomfort that can occur at any time, even during rest). Some patients with the aforementioned criteria may not be candidates for CABG surgery if their left ventricle pumping activity is so poor (25% or less than normal) that their chance of surviving the surgery is low. CABG surgery is also performed in an emergency situation such as when a heart attack is evolving or when angioplasty or the use of "clot-busting" medicines has not been successful.

This operation is performed under general anesthesia and uses a heart-lung machine to support the patient while the surgeon is performing the bypass surgery. The chest is opened (thoracotomy) and the heart is exposed by opening the pericardial sac. This is a "bag" of connective tissue that encloses the heart. The cardiac surgeon identifies the areas along the left and/or right coronary artery that possess the ponderous cholesterol plaques (greater than 70% and generally 90% or more). These are the locations for the bypassing procedure.

The patient is connected to the heart-bypass machine. At this point, the beating heart is stopped, (using a cardioplagic drug), this allows the cardiac surgeon to perform the delicate suturing required. The surgeon then locates the left internal mammary artery. *(Figure 18).* It is usually found alongside the breastbone or sternum and arises from the left subclavian artery. This artery is cut, and the distal (the end portion) segment is tied off. The remaining artery (proximal) is then sutured or sewn into a small opening made by the cardiac surgeon with a scalpel in the left coronary artery (either left anterior descending or circumflex branches) just past the cholesterol plaque.

During this time, another surgeon (vascular surgeon) will be removing a segment of the saphenous vein from the leg of the patient. This is a large vein located under the skin of the leg. Its removal does not cause a problem because there are sufficient numbers of other veins in the leg that will replace its blood-draining function.

The cardiac surgeon will slice the saphenous vein into several segments and prepare them for bypass. A small opening will be made with a scalpel in the ascending aorta, and one end of a saphenous vein will be sutured (medically called anastomosis) to this opening. The other end will be anastomosed (or sutured) to a hole, or incision, made by a scalpel in a coronary artery segment just past a ponderous cholesterol blockage. Several of these anastomoses using saphenous veins can be done *(Figure 19)*. A triple bypass indicates three anastomoses, while a quadruple bypass indicates that four were performed.

When all anastomoses are completed the patient is taken off the heart-bypass machine. Sometimes the heart may be sluggish in starting and the surgeon will use medicines or an electrical shock to "start-up" the heart and allow it to beat normally. The risk of death during this operation is low, approximately 2% or less.

Percutaneous Transmural Coronary Angioplasty (PTCA)

As described in Chapter 3, cardiac catheterization is done to perform coronary angiography which will determine if coronary heart disease is present. However, at times, this procedure allows a doctor to treat the symptoms of coronary heart disease as well. One of the treatments is referred to as balloon percutaneous transmural coronary angioplasty (PTCA), or simply, angioplasty. Balloon angioplasty opens clogged arteries by compressing the cholesterol buildup against the artery wall. To do this, the cardiac catheterization procedure is performed as described in Chapter 3 and a catheter with a small balloon at the end is placed into the introducing tube and moved toward the heart, into the coronary artery, and positioned to where the artery is clogged.

The balloon is inflated and deflated several times in an attempt to compress the cholesterol against the artery wall, opening up the artery and improving the

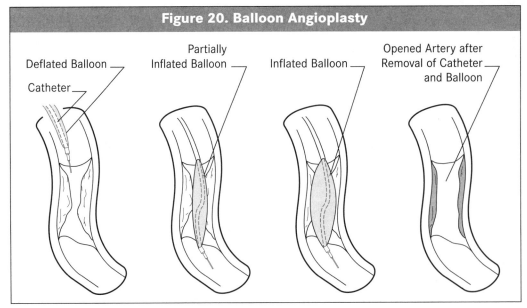

Figure 20. Balloon Angioplasty

Deflated Balloon
Catheter

Partially
Inflated Balloon

Inflated Balloon

Opened Artery after
Removal of Catheter
and Balloon

blood flow *(Figure 20)*. Sometimes, however, the doctor may feel that a stent is necessary. This is because the balloon inflation was not able to keep the artery open. Stents can be lifesaving for patients whose coronary arteries have suddenly closed off during balloon angioplasty due to artery spasm. A spasm closes the coronary artery and may cause a heart attack. A stent is a metal device that in appearance resembles a spring. It is located on the tip of the catheter where a deflated balloon is positioned. When the catheter holding the stent is moved to where the artery is clogged, the balloon is inflated and the stent or spring expands, forcing the cholesterol blockage against the artery wall. The expanded stent is locked and keeps the cholesterol blockage from reforming or entering back into the lumen of the artery *(Figure 21)*.

Both surgical interventions (CABG and PTCA) increase coronary blood flow to the heart muscle and generally alleviate the symptoms of coronary heart disease. This results in an improved quality of daily life and increased exercise capacity, however, does not always guarantee a reduction in the risk of heart attack or death. Only in emergency situations (e.g., during an evolving heart attack or when angioplasty has perforated the coronary artery or caused a spasm) has coronary bypass surgery significantly reduced the risk of death. Also, when the main portion of the left coronary artery is bypassed there is some modest reduction in the risk of death. Yet most of society feels that these procedures partially cure their coronary heart disease and substantially reduce their risk of death, heart

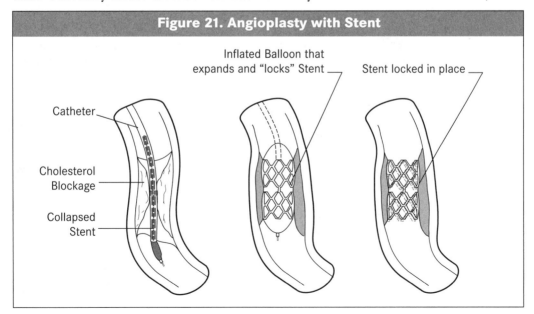

Figure 21. Angioplasty with Stent

Inflated Balloon that expands and "locks" Stent

Stent locked in place

Catheter

Cholesterol Blockage

Collapsed Stent

attack, or need for hospitalization. This is a common misconception that must be clarified. These procedures largely reduce the symptoms, of coronary heart disease, yet do little to reduce the chance of having further complications from this disease.

The reason why these surgical procedures (PTCA and CABG) are not generally effective in improving your chances of survival or reducing your risk of heart attack, is because they treat the wrong cholesterol blockages in the coronary arteries. They treat the blockages that are greater than 70% which are usually durable and not likely to rupture and cause a heart attack. Remember from Chapter 2 that cholesterol blockages occupying 70% or more of the lumen of a coronary artery are durable with thick scar caps over the cholesterol accumulation. They do cause chest discomfort, but generally do not cause heart attack or death because they don't break open and lead to the formation of a blood clot.

During the past five years, a number of clinical studies have been conducted on patients who have had a heart attack. These studies involved people who had coronary angiography within one year before they had the heart attack and then had coronary angiography performed within several days after the heart attack. The x-ray films revealing their blockages in the coronary arteries taken before the heart attack were compared to the x-ray films obtained after the heart attack. These studies revealed where the heart attack occurred, and indicated that it was a "minor" blockage (less than 50%) that prompted the majority of heart attacks. These studies showed that over 85% of all heart attacks occurred at blockage sites of less than 70%, and 60% of all heart attacks occurred at blockages in the coronary arteries of less than 50%.

These studies, which are referred to as "Before and After" studies consistently show that the "culprit blockages," or the blockages that are most likely to cause a heart attack, are generally blocking the coronary artery by less than 50%. Only about 10% of heart attacks occurred at sites in the coronary artery where the blockages exceeded 70%, yet bypass surgery and angioplasty usually address only these blockages. The most threatening blockages, those less than 50%, are not treated by angioplasty or bypass surgery.

When a blockage in a coronary artery is less than 50%, symptoms such as angina may not develop. That is because the coronary artery has the ability to relax (or vasodilate) to an extent where the inside opening increases and blood flow increases, compensating for the partial obstruction. This is a naturally occurring process referred to as autoregulation of blood flow. It is quite likely that a person who has ponderous blockages (greater than 70%) and may receive angioplasty, bypass surgery, or medications such as nitrates, calcium channel blockers, or beta-blockers to reduce the symptoms will also have so-called minor blockages (less than 50%) in their coronary arteries. Cardiologists often refer to these smaller blockages as minor coronary heart disease, or coronary irregularities, which supports the false notion that these are not significant or serious. On the contrary, these are the blockages that are the most vulnerable and likely to cause heart attacks leading to death. (Remember from Chapter 2 that these blockages are quite fragile and can easily break or rupture leading to blood clot formation, stoppage of blood flow and heart attack.)

Treating the Underlying Cause of Coronary Heart Disease— Atherosclerosis

One of the most effective treatments for atherosclerosis, the underlying disease causing coronary heart disease is lowering the blood concentration of LDL-cholesterol. By lowering LDL-cholesterol the atherosclerotic blockages most likely to cause a heart attack are stabilized. Reducing the blood concentration of LDL-cholesterol with subsequent stabilization of atherosclerosis is best accomplished by prudent diet, weight reduction, and medication (specifically statins). The next several pages will attempt to explain to the reader how LDL-cholesterol lowering effectively treats and stabilizes atherosclerotic blockages in the coronary arteries, thereby reducing one's chance of having a heart attack or even dying.

All cholesterol blockages, or atherosclerosis, are composed of cholesterol and varying numbers of white blood cells (remember, white blood cells mediate inflammation) imbedded in the lining of the artery, surrounded by a cap composed of scar tissue (called a fibrous cap). To fully envision the threat of atherosclerosis causing a heart attack, stroke or death, you need to grasp two points. First, you must understand that the cholesterol and inflammation is imbedded in the inner wall of the artery. This means that the cholesterol plaques that are most threatening or likely to cause a heart attack are not those that are mainly above the surface of the inner wall and impinge significantly (greater than 70%) on the opening of the coronary artery. Rather, they are those blockages that are primarily below the surface of the artery wall and in appearance, using coronary angiography, do not seem very alarming because they generally obstruct the opening of the artery by less than 50%.

The second point to understand is that the cap of scar tissue surrounding the embedded cholesterol and inflammation can have varying degrees of thickness. The more severe blockages (70% or greater) tend to have very thick caps. Being thick, these caps are quite sturdy and do not tend to break or crack. However, many of the blockages in the coronary arteries that are less than 50% and have very thin scar caps. They are fragile and are susceptible to breaking open and exposing the underlying cholesterol and inflammation to the blood, causing a blood clot to form which plugs the lumen of the artery. In summary, it is the thickness of the scar cap that determines the degree of stability of a cholesterol plaque, and the thickness of the scar cap is determined by the amount of cholesterol and inflammation that it surrounds.

The reason that less extensive blockages (i.e., less than 50%) have thin scar or fibrous caps is because the white blood cells (macrophages and T-lymphocytes referred to in Chapter 2) below the cap's surface are producing chemical substances (called cytokines and enzymes) that cause inflammation and actually break down the collagen and elastin proteins that render stability and thickness to the scar cap. Therefore, the scar cap thins and becomes fragile, and can easily fracture or tear when plaques contain significant amounts of cholesterol and inflammation. While these less protruding plaques would not seem to be dangerous, they are the ones that most often lead to heart attack and death.

The thickness of the scar cap contributes significantly to the degree that it protrudes into the lumen of the coronary artery. The most obstructive blockages (greater than 70%) tend to have the thickest caps, yet are the safest, relative to not causing a heart attack. The least protruding blockages (less than 50%) tend to have the thinnest caps, are very fragile, and are the most dangerous relative to causing a heart attack.

To better comprehend this point, an analogy of a coronary plaque to an iceberg may be helpful. Some icebergs are quite visible rising out of the water. Naturally, one thinks that the higher it looms, the larger its threat. While this is true to some extent, it is not the whole story on icebergs. The larger the iceberg, the easier it is to detect on the ship's radar and maneuver around it. However, one of the most threatening types of icebergs is the kind that cannot be detected by radar. They do not rise to a great extent above the water. These are called "growlers." While they rise only slightly above the water's surface they are vast just below the surface of the water. Some speculate that it was a growler-type iceberg that was responsible for the Titanic disaster. Atherosclerotic plaques that are most dangerous are like growlers, because as viewed by coronary angiography they appear small and relatively harmless, yet are quite substantial below the inner wall of a coronary artery.

A recently developed technique called Intravascular Ultrasound (IVUS) can assess for the most harmful of vulnerable plaques (blockages) in the coronary arteries. As indicated, coronary angiography shows that these plaques generally protrude into the lumen of a coronary artery by 50% or less. However, IVUS shows that these plaques extend well below the inner wall of the coronary artery and occupy large areas of the middle layer of the artery called the media. IVUS procedures identify vulnerable plaques with their large area of cholesterol in the artery lining and many white blood cells (T-lymphocytes and macrophages) that cause inflammation and weaken the plaque. IVUS is a technique used during a coronary catheterization procedure to assess the vulnerability of plaques and thereby determine risk for rupture and subsequent heart attack risk. At this writing, it is performed in only a few hospitals and medical centers around the country. Dr. Steven E. Nissan, of the Cleveland Clinic Foundation, is a leading authority and expert on the IVUS procedure.

Another test that is receiving significant attention as a potential indicator of the presence of vulnerable or unstable cholesterol blockages/plaques in the coronary arteries is a simple blood test. This test measures the concentration of a substance in the blood called C-reactive protein, or CRP. CRP is produced in the body when inflammation is present. Dr. Paul Ridker of the Harvard Medical School is conducting research that may prove the value of measuring CRP. His research suggests that among patients with coronary heart disease, a high CRP blood concentration predicts future heart attacks. The theory is, since the blockages in the coronary arteries most likely to rupture have large degrees of inflammation associated with them, CRP levels in the blood of these patients would be high. In other words, the higher the blood concentration of CRP, the greater the number of vulnerable plaques and the higher the risk of heart attack. This research is extremely interesting and holds a great deal of promise. However, it is still in the investigational stages and requires additional testing before it can be determined if routine testing for CRP levels in the blood will have genuine value for indicating the presence of vulnerable cholesterol blockages in the coronary arteries. In other words, you should not request the measurement of CRP in your blood from your doctor at this point.

If you have grasped the above concepts, you should presume that the standard medical terms used to describe or label coronary atherosclerotic blockages are very misleading. Basically, they are based upon how much of the blockage can be seen by coronary angiography and consequently, misrepresent how threatening the blockages are to your health and longevity. **I strongly urge you to begin thinking in terms of the new designations listed below:**

Standard Term	Degree of Blockage (per angioplasty)	Risk of Causing a Heart Attack	New Term
Significant or Severe	>70%	Low	Ponderous
Mild	<50%	High	Significant

Aggressive cholesterol lowering (i.e., LDL-cholesterol or "bad" cholesterol) is a highly effective treatment for the blockages that are considered "significant" in our new designation. Studies that have examined the relationship between LDL-cholesterol lowering and subsequent risk of heart attack, death, or hospitalization have shown that reducing the LDL-cholesterol significantly lowers the risk of these coronary events by as much as 40%. Because of the consistency of these findings and the tens of thousands of people participating in these interventional studies, it is generally agreed that LDL is causally related to the formation of atherosclerosis and leads to a high probability of causing a heart attack.

It is clearly evident that by lowering the LDL-cholesterol either with medication, or better, a combination of medication, diet, and weight loss, the cholesterol is slowly dissipated from the lining of the artery wall along with the inflammatory-causing white blood cells, and replaced with scar tissue forming a thicker scar cap. While the percentage of the blockage protruding into the artery lumen may not be significantly changed, the composition of the blockage changes becoming more sturdy and durable. This process is called *plaque stabilization.*

Drug Therapy

The most effective medications for lowering LDL-cholesterol and stabilizing atherosclerosis are the drugs collectively called statins (technically, 3-hydroxy-3-methyl glutaryl-coenzyme A reductase inhibitors). These medicines lower the LDL-cholesterol by inhibiting the production of cholesterol in the liver. When cholesterol production in the liver is reduced, the liver removes LDL from the bloodstream to supply itself with cholesterol for producing bile and making new liver cells. This action reduces LDL-cholesterol concentration in the blood.

Currently there are six prescription statin medicines that are available to physicians for prescribing to patients.

Brand Name	Generic Name
Mevacor	lovastatin
Pravachol	pravastatin
Zocor	simvastatin
Lescol	fluvastatin
Lipitor	atorvastatin
Baycol	cerivastatin

Statin drugs are safe and convenient. They are given once a day, usually at bedtime, and have been proven in controlled, interventional trials to reduce death and morbidity from coronary heart disease among individuals with coronary heart disease. The benefit appears to be independent of the initial LDL-cholesterol concentration in the blood. These clinical trials have also indicated that there is a direct correlation between the degree of reducing LDL-cholesterol and the risk of having a heart attack. The greater the degree of LDL-cholesterol lowering, the greater the clinical benefit. These results again point to the fact that for people with coronary heart disease, target levels of LDL-cholesterol are not as important as reducing the level, no matter what it is. Generally, the interventional studies have shown that an LDL cholesterol reduction from a baseline level of 25% to 35% is necessary to reduce your risk of having of a heart attack by 25% to 35%. Lowering the LDL-cholesterol by 45% below baseline reduces coronary events by about 45%.

Some people fear that lowering their cholesterol or LDL-cholesterol too much may lead to other consequences such as cancer, violent death, or infection. In controlled, interventional studies of cholesterol reduction, these side effects have never been observed. Even in subjects where the LDL-cholesterol levels have been reduced to 60 mg/dL, no increased incidence of cancer or other side effects were observed.

In Chapter 6 you will read the details of the Whitehall and Framingham heart studies, which are survey/observational studies that led some people to believe that low blood cholesterol levels increased the risk of cancer. However, as you will learn, those participating in the study who were found to have cancer, already had the cancer prior to becoming involved in the study. The cancer was not identified at the beginning of these studies so it was assumed that their low cholesterol was causing the cancer. In actuality, it was the undiagnosed cancer taking the cholesterol, primarily the LDL, out of the bloodstream resulting in the low levels of cholesterol. The cancer was the cause of their extremely low cholesterol levels.

It is important to recognize that your body has the capacity to produce the amount of cholesterol that it needs. Therefore, no one with coronary heart disease should be concerned about having too low a cholesterol level as a result of medication and diet. If your body requires cholesterol to manufacture bile or hormones or new cells, it has the ability to manufacture the amount that it needs, even if you are taking a cholesterol-lowering medicine.

Low Saturated Fat Diets

The importance of a prudent diet for people with coronary heart disease will be discussed in greater detail in Chapter 7. However, at this point, a few issues regarding diet need to be mentioned.

The amount of cholesterol that you ingest from the food you eat doesn't significantly determine your blood LDL-cholesterol level. Rather, the amount of dietary saturated fat that you consume does. In other words, while dietary cholesterol is relatively ineffective in raising the concentration of total blood cholesterol or LDL-cholesterol, saturated fats, from dairy products such as cream, whole milk, ice cream, cheese and fatty cuts of beef and pork, and organ meats, are highly effective in raising your LDL-cholesterol. Therefore, diets that work most effectively with cholesterol-lowering drugs are those that restrict your intake of saturated fat to less than 10% of your total daily caloric intake.

When large amounts of saturated fat are ingested, they reduce the ability of the liver to remove LDL from the bloodstream. As a result, the blood level of LDL-cholesterol rises. Since statins reduce blood LDL by increasing the liver's ability to remove it, you can see that if you are taking a statin yet continuing a high saturated fat diet, you run the risk of negating much of the potential benefit of the statin drug. It is important that if you are on a statin drug, you should maintain a diet that ingests no more than 10% of calories from saturated fat (less than 7% is preferred). This will allow the statin drug to work effectively. *(Please refer to Chapter 7 for additional information on diets.)*

Table 1. Cardiovascular Disease Risk Classification Based on Lipids

LDL-Cholesterol	<100mg/dL	Desirable for Patients with Heart Disease
	<130 mg/dlL	Desirable
	130-159 mg/dL	Borderline risk
	≥160 mg/dL	High risk
	≥190 mg/dL	Very high risk
HDL-Cholesterol	<35 mg/dL	Risk factor for men
	<45 mg/dL	Risk factor for women
Triglyceride	<200 mg/dL	Desirable
	200-399 mg/dL	Borderline
	≥400 mg/dL	Risk factor for heart disease
	≥1000 mg/dL	Risk factor for pancreatitis
Total Cholesterol	<200 mg/dL	Desirable
	200-239 mg/dL	Borderline-high levels
	≥240 mg/dL	High levels

Currently, considerable emphasis is placed on the blood cholesterol level, and specifically, the LDL-cholesterol level. The National Cholesterol Education Program sponsored by the federal government has provided guidelines (called the Adult Treatment Panel II Guidelines) regarding lipid, including LDL-cholesterol blood levels.

Many people seem to be under the false impression that a total cholesterol level of 200 mg/dL is important and that if your level is less than 200 mg/dL you are safe from coronary heart disease, whereas if it is over 200 mg/dL you are at increased risk. While this is true for many people **without** coronary heart disease, **it is not true for people** *with* **coronary heart disease**. If you have coronary heart disease it doesn't matter what your total cholesterol or LDL-cholesterol levels are; **they are too high for you.** Doctor Michael S. Brown of Dallas, Texas, who, along with Dr. Joseph Goldstein, won the Nobel prize for Physiology and Medicine in 1985 for their work on understanding LDL function in the body, stated at the 1998 meeting of The American Association of Clinical Chemistry in Chicago, Illinois, "If you have coronary heart disease that means your LDL level is too high no matter what it is."

Your total cholesterol level is not as good a predictor of your risk of developing coronary heart disease or coronary events as is your LDL-cholesterol level. The LDL-cholesterol produces the cholesterol blockages in coronary arteries and can make them susceptible to causing heart attacks. Another major component of the total cholesterol is the HDL-cholesterol, or the good cholesterol. Remember HDL act as scavengers to remove cholesterol from the blood vessel wall. These lipoproteins may help to "stabilize" cholesterol plaques or even prevent them from developing. Therefore, a person may have a high total cholesterol level and wrongly infer that they are at increased risk of coronary heart disease when they are actually not. This would be the case for a person who has a high cholesterol level because the HDL-cholesterol is elevated (i.e., greater than 60 mg/dL).

If you have coronary heart disease your level of LDL-cholesterol is too high for you, no matter what it is. You will reduce the risk of heart attack and death by reducing your LDL-cholesterol. Clinical studies have been conducted among patients with coronary heart disease who have had a wide range of LDL-cholesterol blood concentrations. Even for patients whose blood LDL-cholesterol concentrations are 100 mg/dL or less, treatment with a statin drug lowered their LDL-cholesterol concentrations—and lowered their risk of heart attack, death, and hospitalizations. For people with coronary heart disease LDL-cholesterol or total cholesterol target levels have little significance. For such individuals, their levels are too high for them and they will benefit from reductions.

It seems futile to establish firm target levels of LDL-cholesterol for people with coronary heart disease, because the genetics that control the functions of the coronary arteries are so diverse making a relatively low level of LDL-cholesterol (e.g., 100 mg/dL) dangerous for some and innocuous for others. The ability of LDL to deposit its cholesterol in the lining of an artery requires the sensitivity of the artery wall for allowing this process to occur. Functional properties of the artery wall, like all other functions of the body, are under the control of genes. Many people have inherited "good genes" that make their artery linings somewhat resistant to the negative effects of LDL. There are people who have high levels of LDL-cholesterol and never develop coronary heart disease. For some of these individuals it is likely that their genes make the blood vessel lining resistant to the ability of LDL to deposit cholesterol. By the same token there are a number of people who haven't been so lucky and have inherited genes that result in their arteries being more susceptible to LDL's adverse effects. In these individuals, seemingly favorable levels of LDL-cholesterol (e.g., 100 mg/dL) can lead to cholesterol blockages in the inner coronary artery wall.

Obviously we are all different genetically, yet anyone who has cholesterol blockages in the coronary arteries, or other arteries of the body, has a blood LDL-cholesterol level that is too high. If you have coronary heart disease you should not be obsessed with your total cholesterol or LDL-cholesterol levels. You should just accept that your LDL-cholesterol is too high, regardless of what it is, and you should be following a prudent diet along with taking an LDL-cholesterol lowering drug (i.e., statin). The diet and statin drug will reduce the LDL-cholesterol in your bloodstream, **thereby significantly reducing the impending threat of the existing cholesterol blockages, through making them less likely to lead to a heart attack.** This concept is essentially the take-home message of this book and has been and will continue to be repeated throughout the remaining chapters.

Diabetes Mellitus

Everything that has been recommended concerning the effective treatment of the underlying disease, atherosclerosis, causing coronary heart disease, also applies to patients with diabetes, either with or without coronary heart disease. Recently, the American Diabetes Association has suggested that all diabetics, even in the absence of coronary heart disease, have their LDL-cholesterol and total cholesterol levels treated as if they had coronary heart disease. The reason for this recommendation is because of the results obtained from a recent study conducted in Scandinavia and referred to as The East/West Study. Dr. Stephen Haffner of San Antonio, Texas was a senior investigator and reported the results in the *New England Journal of Medicine* in 1998. This study looked at the risk of having a myocardial infarction or heart attack in four groups of people:

- ▶ people without diabetes and without coronary heart disease
- ▶ people without diabetes but who already had a heart attack (i.e., coronary heart disease)
- ▶ people with diabetes and no evidence of coronary heart disease
- ▶ people who had both coronary heart disease and diabetes

The people were followed for a period of seven years. At the end of the seven years, the risk of having a heart attack in each of the four groups was measured. In the group of patients who were diabetic without coronary heart disease, it was found that their risk of having a heart attack was equal to or greater than the group of people without diabetes who already had one heart attack. This suggests that the presence of diabetes mellitus is a coronary heart disease equivalent.

These results were so compelling to the American Diabetes Association that they recommended that all doctors treat the LDL-cholesterol of diabetics as if they already had coronary heart disease. It is recommended that all diabetics, just as patients with coronary heart disease, take a statin, exercise, and follow a low saturated fat diet. It does not matter what the initial LDL-cholesterol level is, if you have diabetes mellitus lowering your LDL-cholesterol will reduce your risk of heart attack. In addition, it should be noted that coronary heart disease is the major cause of death in diabetics. Nearly 90% of patients with diabetes will die of atherosclerosis (particularly in the coronary arteries) complications.

Conclusion

With all of the proven benefits of LDL-cholesterol-lowering medications (i.e., statins) on coronary heart disease events, stroke, and even death, the fact remains that about half of the people in this country who have coronary heart disease are not receiving these medications along with appropriate diet counseling. Some of the reasons may be because of the misconceptions that people have about these medications. Probably the biggest misconception among people with documented coronary heart disease is that they view cholesterol-lowering medications (statins) as only lowering the total blood cholesterol or LDL-cholesterol levels, when actually, the true value of these medicines is through strengthening, or stabilizing, the most threatening cholesterol blockages in the coronary arteries, making them much less likely to cause a heart attack.

If you are one of the 14 million Americans who have coronary heart disease or 12 million who have diabetes mellitus, you must understand this clearly. The reason you are placed on a cholesterol-lowering medication, such as a statin, is not just to lower the LDL-cholesterol level, but also to treat the atherosclerotic blockages in your coronary arteries that are likely to lead to a heart attack. **The statins make these blockages less vulnerable, less likely to burst, and much less likely to cause a heart attack. That is the primary reason why all 14 million Americans in this country with coronary heart disease (and the 12 million with diabetes) should be on a statin drug along with a prudent diet and exercise, regardless of their baseline LDL-cholesterol level. If you're not on a statin, you should discuss this issue with your doctor.**

The second reason why a significant percentage of people with coronary heart disease do not receive these medications is because they believe the drugs are toxic. This is not true. These are safe medications. You must understand that all medications are foreign to the body and all potentially carry some side effect risk. Statins relative to other medications have a very good safety profile. The press has exaggerated the fact that these medications carry substantial side effects. The actual liver and skeletal muscle side effects that may occur are found in less than 1% of the people who take these medications, and as pointed out, when the medicine is stopped or the dosage reduced, the side effects resolve. *There is no permanent damage.*

The only way that these drugs can cause permanent damage to the liver or to the muscle is if they are taken for a prolonged period of time by a patient who is experiencing liver inflammation or muscle side effects. However, you can protect yourself from this by seeing your doctor every four to six months and having your blood tested for liver and muscle components that can indicate whether you are having an untoward effect.

The most dangerous cholesterol blockages are not those that are visibly obvious by coronary angiography. Additionally, they are generally not the blockages that cause the symptoms (e.g., angina, fatigue, shortness of breath) of coronary heart disease. The blockages that appear the least threatening by angiography (analogy to iceberg growlers) are actually the most threatening to the heart. As the population begins to realize that cholesterol-lowering medications (i.e., statins) stabilize the most dangerous cholesterol plaques, perhaps more and more people who require these medications will take them and take them consistently. Over time, perhaps the general consensus will be that angioplasty and coronary bypass surgery are performed too often in this country. As it stands now, however, the perception of society is that these surgical interventions "cure" heart disease, so these procedures are requested. As people begin to understand that these procedures provide symptomatic relief of coronary heart disease, fewer procedures will be performed and money will be saved.

This is not to say that these procedures are not important. They are very important. Improving the quality of your daily life by relieving the discomfort is necessary and essential. However, when these procedures are performed, they should be done in conjunction with those treatments that treat the underlying disease process. As pointed out, cholesterol-lowering medications such as statins, along with a prudent diet (low saturated fat), treat the blockages that are most likely to lead to heart attack and death. If you are going to put yourself through the discomfort of a bypass procedure, then make sure you are provided with a statin and appropriate dietary recommendations to increase your chances of enjoying and sustaining the symptomatic relief the bypass surgery provided you. And, in the process, increase your chances of prolonging your life.

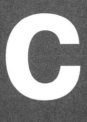

C

Taking Responsibility For Your Cardiovascular Health

Inside Section C:

Chapter 6
Media and Health Studies

As I have suggested, educating yourself about coronary heart disease can be confusing because of a misunderstanding in the distinction between it and other forms of cardiovascular diseases. Also the complexities associated with the causes and complications of this disease can add to the confusion. Hopefully the information in Chapter 2 has provided the reader with a clearer understanding of the various types of cardiovascular disease, and that coronary heart disease is caused by cholesterol build up in the walls of arteries. Chapter 5 should have helped by dispelling several of the myths regarding the traditional ways of treating this disease.

With this better understanding of coronary heart disease, you now have a framework upon which you can build an even greater knowledge and begin to establish a more interactive dialogue with your physician. Also, you are in a position to better evaluate the enormous amount of information disseminated by the media and advertisements regarding how to reduce your risk of acquiring this disease or having further complications.

While the previous chapter (Chapter 5) has summarized many of the approaches to treatment, including the distinction between treatment of the symptoms versus the actual disease process (i.e., atherosclerosis), new treatments are continually being identified and studied, and the results are often published in the medical journals. People are quite eager to learn about new medical breakthroughs and the media will usually attempt to summarize this information (e.g., newspapers, magazines, radio and television reports). Oftentimes, however, the reports are confusing or seemingly conflictive information is reported. This is especially true for coronary heart disease, as well as for other diseases and disorders. (e.g., cancer, arthritis, AIDS, etc.)

One of the most inappropriately used statements by the media or advertisers is, "It has been clinically proven." It is important for you to determine if such a claim is true, or as often is the case, spurious. When you hear or read about a new medical study and its finding, the first thing you must do is to identify whether the results were obtained from a **survey study or an interventional study**. Knowing the distinction is critical to determining if the report is credible or hypothetical. This is not always easy to do. Rarely, if ever, will you hear or read that the particular study was a survey or interventional study. Since the majority of medical studies are survey studies, it's safe for you to assume that most studies reported through the mainstream media are survey studies. These types of studies are oftentimes referred to as cross-sectional studies, case control studies, retrospective studies, epidemiologic studies or longitudinal studies.

Interventional vs. Survey Studies

The difference between the two types of studies is very distinct. An interventional study, as the name implies, involves two or more similar (with respect to age, gender, race, health status, weight, smoking status, etc.) groups of people and some type of intervention or interventions is given to one or more groups. One of the groups of participants serves as a control group and receives a placebo, or sugar pill. The results at the completion of the study can be assessed and compared between the groups, and valid conclusions about the effectiveness and safety of the intervention can be made.

A survey or observational study does not involve an intervention. A survey study follows a group of people and compares differences (e.g., diet, smoking habits, weight, alcohol consumption, etc.) among the people relative to a particular disease outcome, such as coronary heart disease or cancer. Therefore, if you live in a city and hear on the radio that a survey study has recently revealed that coronary heart disease incidence is higher among people living by a busy street, before you put your house up for sale and move to the country, you need to determine a few details about the study. For instance, you need to know where the study was conducted and whether or not it was near a toxic waste dump or chemical plant. Did all of the streets where the people lived share similar characteristics, such as increased traffic flow? Were the people generally older, or middle aged? Was there a higher prevalence of smokers than the national average? You need to determine the socioeconomic circumstances and other issues concerning the people participating in the study. In essence, survey studies can be fraught with a number of issues that could directly or indirectly influence the results. In the above example, the stress associated with living near a busy street in a city may have had absolutely nothing to do with the higher incidence of coronary heart disease. The social traits (e.g., diet, smoking or drinking habits), age (older vs. younger citizens), or environmental influences (heavy exhaust fumes from the vehicles) may have been the culprits. Results from survey studies must be viewed with some skepticism, because their purpose is not to identify cause and effect. Their purpose is to identify associations and formulate hypotheses or theories that will require validation.

This is not to imply that results from a survey study are not helpful. Survey studies do serve useful purposes. As pointed out they generate hypotheses or theories. They also help identify risk factors associated with a disease or disorder. A risk factor does not necessarily mean a causal factor; rather it is simply a trait (e.g., gender, excess body weight, etc.) or habit (e.g., sedentary life style), that is more often observed among individuals with a particular disease than individuals without that disease. Identification of a risk factor would then need to be evaluated in an interventional study to determine if it is causally related to a disease. For example, a high blood concentration of C-reactive protein (CRP) has been identified as a risk factor for heart attack in survey studies (Chapter 5). Remember, Dr. Paul Ridker of the Harvard Medical School found higher concentrations of CRP in the blood of people who went on to have heart attacks. However, this observation does not prove that elevated CRP concentrations *cause* heart attacks. To validate this risk factor as causal, one would need to identify thousands of people with high CRP blood levels and randomize half to a medicine that reduces CRP and half to a placebo. The study participants would then be followed for several months to years and tracked for heart attack and other coronary events. If after this period of time, there were significantly fewer heart attacks in the participants receiving the medicine that lowered blood CRP levels compared to those receiving the placebo, then it could be said that CRP contributes to heart attack and its reduction would be of benefit. Results from interventional studies provide the basis for evidence-based medicine, and thereby their results are generally applicable to the population at large.

Using results from survey studies to direct treatment of a particular disease or to reduce the risk of developing a disease can be risky. To highlight this point through a real example, consider the survey studies evaluating the impact of hormone replacement therapy in on coronary heart disease in postmenopausal females. Numerous survey studies have indicated that hormone replacement, particularly estrogen, seems to help protect postmenopausal women from cardiovascular disease. The majority of these survey (i.e., epidemiologic) studies have clearly found this association. These studies observed less coronary heart disease among post menopausal women taking hormone replacement therapy than those not taking hormones. Therefore, it was commonplace for many years to consider hormone replacement therapy for a postmenopausal female as a way to reduce her risk of cardiovascular disease, particularly coronary heart disease.

Because of these consistent results from the survey studies, the HERS trial (Heart Estrogen/Progestin Replacement Study), an interventional study examining the effect of hormone replacement therapy on cardiovascular disease, was conducted in order to validate the survey study observations. The results of the HERS trial were published in 1998 in the *Journal of the American Medical Association* by Dr. Stephen Hulley of San Francisco and his associates. This study took a group of over 2,700 postmenopausal females who all had a history of coronary heart disease. Some had prior heart bypass surgery or angioplasty, and others had a prior heart attack or a confirmed (by coronary angiography) diagnosis of coronary heart disease. None of these women were receiving hormone replacement therapy. At the start of the study, half of the women were given estrogen and a small dose of progestin, and the other half a placebo or sugar pill. (To reduce the risk of estrogen-associated endometrial cancer, doctors routinely include progestins with hormone replacement regimens for postmenopausal women who have not had a hysterectomy.)

The women were followed for five years. At the end of the five-year period, cardiovascular disease including manifestations of coronary heart disease (heart attack, need for heart bypass surgery) were examined between the two groups. No difference was found in any of these outcomes between the women who received the hormones versus those who received the sugar pill. In addition, when the results were examined on a yearly basis, it was observed that the women who received the hormones had, in the first year, a significantly higher incidence of heart attack than those women who received the sugar pill. Also, the women receiving the hormones had a higher incidence of gallbladder disease and blood clotting events than those receiving the placebo.

These results are quite alarming considering the fact that it was generally perceived (based on survey studies) that hormone replacement therapy protects women from cardiovascular disease. This is an example of the dangers of assuming that the results of a survey study establish cause and effect and therefore, should be applied to the treatment of a disease or to lower the risk of a disease. Because of the HERS trial results, initiation of hormone replacement therapy is not recommended for postmenopausal women with coronary heart disease. If a postmenopausal woman is taking hormones and develops coronary heart disease, the decision whether to continue the hormones should be made on an individual basis by the woman and her doctors (i.e., cardiologist and ob/gyn).

Currently, there is an ongoing interventional study called The Women's Health Initiative—a multicenter study being conducted in medical schools, hospitals and health centers across the country—which will better indicate the role of hormone replacement therapy for providing a cardiovascular benefit to postmenopausal women. At this point, any woman considering hormone replacement therapy should discuss the issue completely with her gynecologist or primary care physician. The risks and potential benefits must be weighed. Until additional information from interventional studies is obtained (i.e., Women's Health Initiative results), hormone replacement therapy in postmenopausal women for cardiovascular risk reduction must be made on a case by case basis with the woman's physician. No general guideline can be made at this time.

While many observational studies have found that there are several risk factors associated with the coronary heart disease, cause and effect based on the results from interventional studies have been established for only a few of these risk factors, namely smoking and LDL-cholesterol. The modifiable risk factors that have been found to be associated with an increased risk of coronary heart disease, but have not been officially established as causally related, include obesity, sedentary lifestyle, Type A personality, and elevated concentrations of triglycerides, CRP, and homocysteine. Also, hypertension (high blood pressure) and diabetes mellitus have not been clearly established as causal for coronary heart disease. Bear in mind, these factors have generally been found to be associated with the disease—not the causes of its development.

The Framingham Study

A good example of an observational study that looked at coronary heart disease and risk factors is the Framingham Heart Study. The Framingham Heart Study began in 1949 in Framingham, Massachusetts. Its purpose was to follow residents living in the Framingham area for long periods of time and observe differences among those who developed cancer or coronary heart disease compared to those that remained free of these chronic diseases.

Factors that were examined in these people included smoking habits, diabetes mellitus, blood cholesterol levels, and blood pressure. After various periods of time (five years, ten years, and fifteen years), these factors in the individuals who developed cancer or coronary heart disease were looked at and compared to these factors in individuals who remained free of these diseases. What was observed was that those individuals who developed cancer had a higher incidence of smoking and obesity, while those who developed coronary heart disease had a higher prevalence of high cholesterol and triglycerides, hypertension, smoking, obesity, and diabetes. However, to determine cause and effect of any of these risk factors, controlled interventional trials were required. Some of these interventional studies have been completed.

Of those identified risk factors for coronary heart disease, elevated cholesterol (specifically LDL-cholesterol) has undergone the most rigid and reproducible evaluations and has been established as a causal factor for coronary heart disease. There have been six recent, large (4,000 to 9,000 participants per study) controlled interventional studies conducted on the benefits of LDL-cholesterol reduction on coronary events. The four studies listed below involved patients with diagnosed coronary heart disease at the beginning of each study and therefore, make them relevant to this book.

► The Scandinavian Simvastatin Survival Study ("4S")
► Cholesterol and Recurrent Events Trial ("CARE Trial")
► Post Coronary Artery Bypass Grafting Study ("Post-CABG Study")
► Lipid Intervention with Pravastatin in Ischemic Disease Study ("LIPID Study")

The other two studies will be relevant to my next book, *The ABC's of Preventing Coronary Heart Disease*. They were conducted among subjects who did not have evidence of coronary heart disease at the beginning of the studies.

► West of Scotland Coronary Prevention Study (WOSCOPS)
► Air Force/Texas Coronary Atherosclerosis Prevention Study (AF/Tex CAPS)

Should you review the interventional studies listed, you will see that all of them have consistently demonstrated a beneficial effect of lowering LDL-cholesterol on coronary heart disease. If, on the other hand, you examined the survey or observational studies pertaining to cholesterol and cardiovascular disease, you would notice that not all of them show an association between high blood cholesterol levels and coronary heart disease.

Remember, in an interventional trial, the researcher or investigator intervenes in some way in one group of individuals versus another group, and then follows them for the development of a particular outcome, such as coronary heart disease. The investigation also *randomizes* participants to a control group and to an interventional group, in an attempt to balance, between the two groups, other potential contributing factors to coronary heart disease (e.g., smoking status, age, gender, prevalence of diabetes and hypertension). In the case of LDL-cholesterol, a number of interventional studies (listed above) have confirmed that, by intervening with diet and drugs to lower the LDL-cholesterol, coronary heart disease and its complications are markedly reduced. The studies all clearly demonstrate that, for every 1% that you lower your blood LDL-cholesterol level, you reduce your risk of having a fatal or nonfatal coronary event by 1%. Therefore, the greater you lower the LDL-cholesterol, the greater you reduce your risk of having a coronary event. The consistency of this finding among these studies clearly establishes LDL-cholesterol as causally related to coronary heart disease.

In addition, these studies also showed that lowering the LDL-cholesterol reduced stroke events and all causes of death. This latter effect is an important point. It demonstrates that it is a misconception to think that by lowering blood cholesterol, specifically LDL-cholesterol, you increase your risk of contracting another serious disease, such as cancer. As mentioned in Chapter 4, increased risk of cancer was not at all observed in any of the clinical interventional studies of LDL-cholesterol lowering.

The Whitehall Study

The reason that many people believe that low blood cholesterol levels may cause cancer is because of the results from an observational (survey) study. Specifically, this was an observational study conducted in the Whitehall District of London, England. This study looked at blood levels of total cholesterol in a group of people living in London, England, and related them to all causes of death over an eight year period. They found that those individuals who had low levels of total cholesterol (less than 140 mg/dL) had a higher incidence of cancer mortality than expected. People in this study who had elevated total cholesterol levels (generally greater than 200 mg/dL) had a high incidence of death from coronary heart disease. The assumption was made that there was a causal link between low blood cholesterol and cancer. This was an inappropriate assumption to make because survey studies are not suitable for establishing cause and effect. However, the Whitehall study results were reported in newspapers as evidence that low blood cholesterol levels cause cancer.

A close examination of the data from the Whitehall survey (epidemiological) study revealed several interesting points. The relationship between the extremely low levels of cholesterol and cancer occurred only during the first year of follow-up of the study. In the second year and beyond, there was no relationship between low cholesterol and cancer. The medical records of the individuals who developed cancer in the first year and had very low cholesterol levels, revealed that many of them had undiagnosed cancers at the time of enrollment in the study. We all know that cancer cells are rapidly growing and they have a great need for cholesterol from LDL to allow for their cells to grow. Remember, cholesterol is a structural component of cell membranes.

What actually happened in this study is that those individuals who had undetected cancers had lower cholesterol levels because the tumors and the tumor cells were pulling the LDL-cholesterol out of the bloodstream, causing their levels to be low. In interventional studies like those listed earlier, where total cholesterol, and specifically LDL-cholesterol, levels were lowered to extremely low concentrations (i.e., total cholesterol levels less than 140 mg/dL, LDL-cholesterol levels less than 60 mg/dL), no increased cancer was ever observed. The point of all of this is that no one should be concerned that low cholesterol can increase the risk of cancer. As pointed out earlier, the body will produce the cholesterol it needs.

The Whitehall study is another excellent example of the flaw in making cause and effect relationships from survey or observational studies. This is especially obvious if you critically analyze how the data was interpreted. Furthermore, the Whitehall study shows the impact of the overeagerness of skeptics and the media when it comes to publicizing new, shocking, or alternative information regarding medical studies and their findings.

In summary, lower blood levels of LDL-cholesterol are associated with less cardiovascular death. The interventional studies that have lowered LDL-cholesterol in a variety of people have found reductions in the complications produced by coronary heart disease, including the need for heart bypass surgery, hospitalizations for unstable angina, heart attacks, strokes, and mortality. The people involved in these studies were those with coronary heart disease, those without, those with extremely high total cholesterol levels, and those with normal or low total cholesterol levels. Regardless of the presence or absence of coronary heart disease, and regardless of the baseline total cholesterol level, everyone benefits from lowering their LDL-cholesterol relative to the risk of developing coronary heart disease or having recurrent problems should the disease be present. **If you have coronary heart disease, you should be taking a statin (cholesterol-lowering drug), following a low saturated fat diet, and exercising (of course, stop smoking if you are a smoker!) no matter what your total cholesterol or LDL-cholesterol levels are. Lower is better**.

Conclusion

Survey studies (epidemiological, case-control, cross-sectional, retrospective, etc.) only establish associations between variables and a particular outcome. The results are useful for initiating hypotheses or for identifying risk factors. *They do not establish cause and effect.* The best way to determine if a study is survey or interventional is by identifying if an intervention (e.g., drug, diet, surgical procedure, etc.) was administered to some of the study participants while others in the study served as a control group. If you have determined that you are reading about the results obtained from a survey study, you should not take this information as the gospel truth. You should recognize that it is only an observation and may not necessarily be applicable to you. It is best to ignore the results of such a study and use your own good judgment, or better yet, discuss it with your physician.

However, if you are reading about the results from an interventional study, you can assure yourself that the information is most likely reliable. Remember, in interventional studies the groups of participants are generally identical in every way (i.e., age distribution, proportions of men and women, racial differences) except that one group receives an active intervention and the other group receives a placebo or sugar pill. In other words, the only difference between the groups is the *intervention* being studied. Should the group that received the intervention have a different outcome from the control group, you can be reasonably assured that cause and effect has been established and that there is a benefit (or in some cases, a detriment) to receiving whatever intervention was used in the study.

The validity of interventional trials for proving cause and effect is so high that the Food and Drug Administration (FDA) requires pharmaceutical companies to conduct them to determine the effectiveness and **safety** of investigational drugs. Only upon proving effectiveness and safety through well-controlled interventional studies will the FDA approve a drug for use. Basically, if you follow the rule that survey study results are oftentimes suspect and interventional study results are generally accurate, it will become much easier for you to make the right judgments about medical studies being reported in the media.

If you are a member of the media, please take the time to determine whether or not the information you are reporting is based on either a survey/observational study or an interventional study. One of the greatest services that both the media and physicians can do for the people in the United States is to educate them about the difference between these two types of studies. Once educated, they can make better decisions about their health, and more effectively interact with their doctors and other health care professionals.

References for the trials listed in this chapter

▶ 4 (S): *The Lancet,* Vol. 344, pages 1383-1389, 1994.

▶ CARE: *New England Journal of Medicine,* Vol. 335, pages 1001-1009, 1996.

▶ Post-CABG: *New England Journal of Medicine,* Vol. 336, pages 153-162, 1997 and *American Journal of Cardiology,* Vol. 82, pages 45T-48T, 1998.

▶ LIPID: *New England Journal of Medicine,* Vol. 339, pages 1349-1357, 1998.

Chapter 7
Diet

If you recall from Chapter 5, the fundamental principle regarding diet for a person with coronary heart disease is to limit your intake of saturated fats—which come from primarily dairy products and fatty cuts of beef, pork and organ meats—to less than 10% of your total calories. Actually, it is preferable to reduce your saturated fat intake to less than 7% of your total daily caloric intake. Your objective is to lower your blood level of LDL-cholesterol and allow the cholesterol-lowering medicine to achieve its maximal effectiveness. Reducing your saturated fat intake helps the medicine to impact your liver to remove LDL from the bloodstream. When you ingest large amounts of saturated fats, you hinder your liver's ability to do this and consequently counteract the effectiveness of the cholesterol-lowering medicine and your blood LDL-cholesterol level rises.

American Heart Association and National Cholesterol Education Program Diets

The American Heart Association and the National Cholesterol Education Program Diets recommend that all individuals maintain good cardiovascular health with a low fat diet. These diets are comprised of two steps:

Step I—recommended for anyone over the age of two.
Step II—recommended for adults who have coronary heart disease or other atherosclerotic diseases such as stroke or claudication.

Table 2 indicates the essential elements of these diets.

Table 2. Elements of Step I and Step II Low Fat Diets		
Element	Step I Diet	Step II Diet
Calories	A level to achieve or maintain desirable weight	Same
Total fat	30% or less of calories	Same
Saturated fat	8% to 10% of calories	Less than 7% of calories
Polyunsaturated fat	Up to 15% of calories	Same
Monounsaturated fat	Up to 15% of calories	Same
Carbohydrate (sugar)	55% or more of calories	Same
Protein	About 15% of calories	Same
Cholesterol	Less than 300 mg per day	Less than 200 mg per day

Both diets reduce the total caloric intake from fat to under 30% of daily consumed calories and are designed to lower the blood LDL-cholesterol level. The Step II diet is more saturated fat- and cholesterol-restrictive than the Step I diet and is therefore better suited for coronary heart patients. The Step II diet reduces a person's intake of saturated fat to less than 7% of daily calories, and cholesterol to under 200 milligrams (mg) per day. Common dietary sources of saturated fat are:

> animal fats—fatty cuts of meat (beef, pork, lamb, organ meats, & poultry)
> specific plant oils—palm, coconut, & palm kernel oils
> dairy products—butter, milk, cream, cheese, sour cream, ice cream, & eggs (egg yolk is the most concentrated source of dietary cholesterol)
> processed cakes, cookies, crackers and snack foods

Successful adherence to this diet requires reading the labels of food products and a little knowledge of arithmetic. Fat, sugar and protein provide the body with energy, or fuel, to operate successfully. The amount of energy per gram of each of these nutrients is indicated in the following formula:

1 gram of protein = 4 calories (of energy)
1 gram of sugar= 4 calories
1 gram of fat= 9 calories

Based on this information, you can calculate the number of calories of fat, sugar and protein from a food source and the percentage of the total number of calories for each nutrient.

The best way to demonstrate this is with an example. Let's determine the percentage of calories for each nutrient in an 8-ounce carton of skim milk. The label reads as follows:

protein: 8 grams
sugar: 12 grams
fat: 0 grams

Total calories: 80

You perform the following calculation:

protein: 8 grams x 4 calories = 32 calories
sugar: 12 grams x 4 calories = 48 calories
fat: 0 grams x 9 calories = 0 calories

% of protein calories: 32/80 x 100 = 40%
% of sugar calories: 48/80 x 100 = 60%
% of fat calories: 0/80 x 100 = 0%

The above information can be used to calculate the percentage of protein, sugar, and fat for an entire day's food consumption. Your doctor or registered dietician can help you to determine the total number of calories you should consume per day to achieve or maintain a good body weight.

Generally, the calories needed to maintain one pound of body weight is based, in part, on your activity level. The following is a good "rule of thumb" to follow for identifying your daily caloric intake:

Activity Level	Calories Required per Pound
Sedentary	10
Light Activity (housework)	13
Active (moderate exercise 3X/week)	15
Heavy Exercise (aerobic exercise 6X/week, manual labor)	18

The following are examples of how to calculate the number of calories per day to be consumed to achieve or maintain a particular body weight:

Example 1: 40 year old female, weighing 140 pounds, **active** and would like to achieve a body weight of 125 pounds.

125 pounds x 15 calories = 1,875 calories per day

She would need to continue her active lifestyle and reduce her daily caloric consumption to 1,875 calories per day to achieve and maintain a body weight of 125 pounds.

Example 2: 50 year old male, weighing 200 pounds, **light activity**, and wants to achieve a body weight of 160 pounds.

160 pounds x 13 calories = 2,080 calories per day is required

It is quite easy to estimate the number of calories of food to be consumed per day to achieve or maintain a particular body weight. Remember that your activity level is important.

The Step II diet recommended by the American Heart Association and National Cholesterol Education Program for patients with coronary heart disease is designed to help lower the LDL-cholesterol blood level and body weight (if necessary) through adjusting the total caloric intake. There are however, other diets that heart patients have read about and may consider adopting. The most popular are the Mediterranean diet and the Atkins' diet.

The Mediterranean Diet

While all of us are sensitive to saturated fat, that is, it raises the blood concentration of LDL-cholesterol, some of us are also sensitive to carbohydrate or sugar. This means that some people who consume foods low in fat, substitute carbohydrate (and oftentimes, excessively) for fat calories, and this will lead to weight gain. A rise in the blood concentration of triglycerides with a reduction in the HDL-cholesterol level also will occur. A diet that is well suited for these individuals, as well as people with coronary heart disease is the "Mediterranean Diet."

The term "Mediterranean Diet" has a specific meaning. It is not a true diet as much as it is a style of eating. It is a way of eating that reflects the dietary habits of the people living in Greece, Crete, and southern Italy during the early to mid 1960s. This time period and geographical location is based on the following:

1. Adult life expectancy for people living in this geographical area was among the highest in the world. The prevalence of coronary heart disease and certain forms of cancer were very low.

2. Information about the dietary habits and food intake of the people living in this area demonstrated consistency and similarity.

3. Similar dietary patterns and food consumption have been associated with low rates of coronary heart disease and high adult life expectancy in several epidemiological studies conducted throughout the world.

A diet reflective of the eating habits of the people living in this region of the Mediterranean during the 1960s had the following characteristics:

1. 25% to 35% of total calories from fat (less than 7% of calories from saturated fat)

2. 20% to 25% of calories from protein

3. 45% to 50% of calories from carbohydrate

This represents a diet similar to the American Heart Association or National Cholesterol Education Program Step II diets (i.e., less than 7% of calories from saturated fat), yet is different, in that a Mediterranean diet provides more mono- and polyunsaturated fats, a little more protein, and *a lesser amount of carbohydrate or sugar.*

Essentially, the general characteristics of a Mediterranean approach to one's diet include the following principles:

1. A significant amount of food from plant sources (vegetables, nuts, whole grain breads and cereals, beans, and fresh fruits). Nuts, such as almonds, are a healthy source of protein.

2. Very minimal consumption of processed foods (cakes, cookies, lunch meats, crackers, frozen dinners). Fresh fruit is consumed as a typical dessert.

3. Olive oil is a primary source of fat. It should be used in salad dressings, food preparation, and as an alternative to butter or margarine spreads on bread.

4. Honey is substituted for sugar.

5. Moderate daily consumption of fish and to a lesser degree poultry.

6. Low consumption of dairy products. Dairy products consumed are principally white cheeses and yogurt.

7. Low consumption of lean red meats (beef, pork and lamb).

8. Zero to four eggs per week.

9. Wine is consumed in small quantities and primarily with meals.

A Mediterranean diet pyramid *(Figure 22)* depicts the types and frequencies of servings of foods and food groups that contribute to this style of eating.

The reasons that the patterns and type of food consumption were so characteristic of the region during the 1960s are quite interesting. Dairy products were minimally consumed because refrigeration was lacking and the climate was frequently hot. Milk in the Mediterranean region was preserved and consumed as yogurt and cheese. Fish was consumed over red meat because of the availability from the Mediterranean Sea. Olive oil was the region's principal source of fat because of tradition established over two to three thousand years. The abundance of fresh vegetables, nuts, olives and seeds led to their incorporation as major staples of the diets of the Mediterranean people. Wine consumption in low to moderate amounts has been a tradition for hundreds of years for people living in

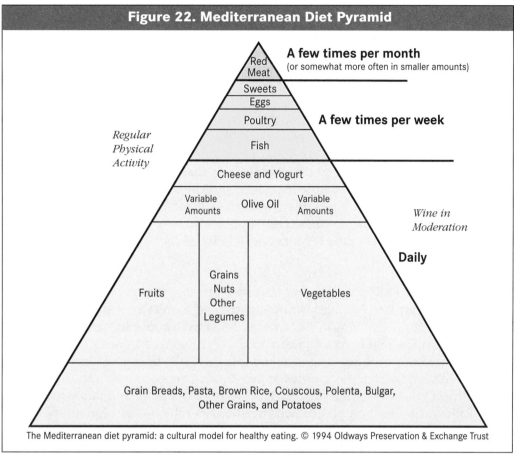

Figure 22. Mediterranean Diet Pyramid

A few times per month
(or somewhat more often in smaller amounts)

Red Meat

Sweets

Eggs

Poultry

A few times per week

Fish

Regular Physical Activity

Cheese and Yogurt

Variable Amounts

Olive Oil

Variable Amounts

Wine in Moderation

Daily

Fruits

Grains Nuts Other Legumes

Vegetables

Grain Breads, Pasta, Brown Rice, Couscous, Polenta, Bulgar, Other Grains, and Potatoes

The Mediterranean diet pyramid: a cultural model for healthy eating. © 1994 Oldways Preservation & Exchange Trust

Greece and southern Italy. It is consumed primarily with family meals and often-times mixed with water.

When the Mediterranean diet is consumed in appropriate and sufficient amounts, it provides all of the known essential nutrients and micronutrients (i.e., vitamins and minerals). It also provides an appropriate amount of fiber and fiber helps to lower the blood concentration of LDL-cholesterol. This diet constitutes thousands of years of tradition and contributes to good health and provides a sense of pleasure and well-being. While the diet pyramid describes the traditional diet, it can be easily adapted through appropriate food exchanges to fit the American way of life.

Recently, a controlled interventional study using the Mediterranean diet was conducted in individuals with coronary heart disease. The study was called the Lyon Diet Heart Study. It was a randomized, single-blind, secondary prevention (that is, conducted in people with known coronary heart disease) trial, aimed at testing whether a Mediterranean-type diet, compared with a **prudent** western diet, reduces the recurrence of coronary events. It concluded that individuals following a Mediterranean-like diet did have reductions in all of the following: plasma, LDL-cholesterol and triglycerides, as well as heart attacks and hospitalization, compared to those following the prudent Westernized diet (i.e., similar to the American Heart Association recommended diet). Remember the Mediterranean-like diet is a good alternative to the low fat diet of the American Heart Association, if you have coronary heart disease. It is especially appropriate if you are "sugar sensitive" or need to lose weight. A visit to your registered dietician will provide you with meal menus that include fish, olive and canola oils, nuts and other good protein sources without significant amounts of saturated fats (e.g., egg whites, low fat yogurt, skim milk, soy beverage). A glass or two of wine per day is also included, along with vegetables, fruits and whole grains.

The Atkins' Diet

The Atkins' diet is a high protein and fat, low sugar diet that is very different from the Mediterranean diet. Popularly known as the "high protein" diet, the Atkins' diet has received a lot of attention because of its effectiveness in quickly reducing body weight. It is a diet composed of about 40% to 45% of calories from protein, about 40% to 45% of calories from fat, and less than 10% of calories from sugar (or carbohydrates). However, the sources of protein that are recommended in this diet are also high in saturated fats such as found in fatty meats and dairy products. If you follow this diet, you may experience considerable weight loss initially. This weight loss is believed to come from the loss of body water and the greater satiety (i.e., feeling of fullness) value of substituting protein and fat for carbohydrate. In addition, after a period of time, the diet causes a loss of appetite due to the accumulation of ketones in the body (called ketosis), a chemical by-product manufactured in the body as a result of metabolizing fat instead of carbohydrates.

For a variety of reasons, this diet has been viewed skeptically by the medical community. There are a number of potential long-term consequences of this diet, including the increased risk of developing kidney stones, gout, vitamin B deficiency, and advances in kidney failure, particularly in diabetics. Several physicians have observed that patients who follow the Atkins' diet, while experiencing weight reduction in the first two months, see marked elevations of LDL-cholesterol in their bloodstream. Specifically, Dr. John C. LaRosa,[2] while a professor at the George Washington University Medical Center, and his associates, clearly showed

---

[2] Dr. LaRosa's study was published in the *Journal of the American Dietetic Association*, Vol. 77, pages 264 to 270, 1980.

that this diet raises the blood concentration of LDL-cholesterol. Again, the high saturated fat intake impairs the ability of the liver to remove LDL, which leads to an LDL-cholesterol increase in the bloodstream. As a result, the risk for coronary heart disease also increases.

Dr. LaRosa's study showed that in the initial weeks of the diet, the rapid weight reduction brought about a reduction in the plasma triglyceride concentration. After several weeks there was a marked rise in the LDL-cholesterol concentration of about 20%. The "good" cholesterol level (HDL) dropped by 12% in women. This drop in HDL was surprising because of the weight reduction achieved. Normally, weight reduction raises HDL-cholesterol. Since it drops with the Atkins' diet, this suggests that the composition of the diet (i.e., high saturated fat and protein intake) has detrimental effects on HDL. Blood uric acid levels also increased as the result of this diet.

These changes in LDL-cholesterol and HDL-cholesterol seen in people following the Atkins' diet will increase the risk of atherosclerosis several fold. Additionally, the uric acid level increase can lead to heightened risk of gout (uric acid increased by 25%). *Therefore, because this diet increases your chances of acquiring or complicating coronary heart disease, it is not recommended for patients with coronary heart disease, or for that matter, anyone, as a means of losing weight.*

The Adkins' diet is considered one of many diets referred to as "fad diets." Fad diets should be avoided by people with coronary heart disease because they generally lack proven effectiveness and **may be harmful**. There are several warning signs that you should be aware of when reading or hearing about a particular diet that promises benefits that are likely too good to be true.

Warning Signs:
- diet recommendations promise a "quick fix"
- recommendations based on survey (observational) studies or a single interventional study
- diet that lists good and bad foods
- impressive claims that are refuted by medical societies or reputable scientific organizations
- recommendations made to help sell nutritional products

Conclusion

Not only is diet important for allowing cholesterol-lowering medications to work effectively, it is also important for weight reduction. **Medical study after medical study has clearly and consistently demonstrated that body leanness is associated with good health and longevity.** As we get older we need less food, rather than more food. Even though our body seemingly craves food, that is, you are experiencing hunger pangs, this does not mean that it requires food. You may just be thirsty, so try drinking a 10-ounce glass of water first before you eat a snack or a meal. Either your thirst (which may have been deceiving you into thinking you were hungry) or your hunger will be satisfied, without excess calories. This is a very effective dieting or weight management technique; **drink a 10-ounce glass of water before each meal and snack.**

You also have to acknowledge to yourself the fact that like most of us, you may eat excessively because of habit. That is, many of us are food-addicted to some extent in much the same way as people are addicted to cigarettes, alcohol, or drugs. Our bodies have been conditioned over a period of time to eat fatty foods or sugars, to eat in excess, for comfort, or before going to bed, and it is hard to break these habits. When we try to break these habits our bodies respond with withdrawal symptoms such as excessive hunger pangs, irritability, even light-headedness. If you have coronary heart disease you have to make the effort along with your doctor to reduce your risk of dying or having a heart attack. That effort includes changing your behavior patterns toward nutrition and diet. **There are no magic pills.**

It is imperative that if you have coronary heart disease you meet at least once with a registered dietician. A registered dietician can provide you menus that adhere to the guidelines of a low fat diet or the Mediterranean diet. The dietician will also help you make appropriate food substitutions so that you can enjoy more of the foods you like. Determining portion sizes is also an important consideration that the dietician will assist you with, particularly if you need to lose weight. I recommend the Mediterranean diet over the American Heart Association low fat diet, because the former has less sugar and higher amounts of the heart-healthy fats (i.e., monounsaturated fats) and protein. A diet similar to the Mediterranean diet is the so-called Zone diet. This is a diet that recommends approximately one-third of calories from carbohydrates, (i.e., sugars) one-third from protein, and one third from fat. **The key to any healthy diet is a reduction in saturated fat.**

If you have coronary heart disease you should not be consuming more than 10% of your calories from saturated fat. Actually, no more than 7% of calories is preferred. It is best to increase your intake of protein to about 25% of calories, remembering that the protein sources often accompany fat. Therefore, stay away from fatty meats (as promoted by the Atkins' diet) and focus on protein sources that are accompanied by good fats such as fish, nuts (peanuts, walnuts, almonds), soy products, and egg whites. For example, almonds have as much protein as an ounce of red meat and do not have as much saturated fat. They have monounsaturated fats that will raise the blood level of HDL-cholesterol. Almonds also are a good source of the antioxidant vitamin E.

Reduction in simple sugars means not only candies, cakes, and sweets, but also, sweet fruits. Avoid starches that lead to formation of simple sugars in the body such as pastas, white breads and white rice. When eaten in excess, they can result in weight gain.

In short, a practical diet and maintaining your body's appropriate weight is essential for allowing cholesterol-lowering (statins) drugs to work optimally. That is lowering the blood LDL-cholesterol and stabilizing the plaques in your coronary arteries. This will reduce your risk of having a heart attack or dying. Remember, studies have shown that diet and cholesterol-lowering medications will also reduce your risk of stroke. **Eating the proper foods is one of the most effective lifestyle adjustments that you can make. Eating a variety of food provides the vitamins, minerals, nutrients, and fiber that we all need to maintain good health. "Variety is the spice of life." Remember, monitoring the quantity you eat is important.**

Chapter 8
Vitamins and Nutritional Supplements

One of the principal themes of this book is how important it is for you to take responsibility for your health, especially if you have been diagnosed with coronary heart disease. Even if you have already had a heart attack, undergone heart bypass surgery or angioplasty, or if you are experiencing angina, there are measures you can take that can enhance your quality of life and help reduce your risk of a future heart attack or sudden death. This chapter is dedicated to informing you of what you can do for yourself, in addition to the recommendations and therapy provided by your doctor and other health care professionals (i.e., medication and diet).

The newspapers, magazines, television and radio broadcasts are saturated with advertisements and reports about vitamins, nutritional supplements, alcohol, specific foods and "fad" diets that are touted to lower your LDL-cholesterol concentration or reduce your risk of coronary heart disease and its complications. With that in mind, you need to know how you can impact your cardiovascular health through the value or possible dangers of heeding the recommendations thrown at you by the manufacturers or sponsors of products and diets commercially designed to "improve health." Each recommendation or discouragement I make in this chapter has been arrived at through evidence-based medicine (i.e., the results of interventional studies published in peer-reviewed medical journals).

Vitamins and Nutritional Supplements

Vitamins, nutritional supplements, and herbs have become very popular over the past decade as a means of maintaining good health and preventing all sorts of diseases, including coronary heart disease. The manufacturers of nutritional supplements and herbs have certainly helped spawn their popularity by suggesting that their products can help you lower your cholesterol or reduce your risk of coronary heart disease by "natural" means as opposed to medicines which carry substantial "side effect" risks. Through their very effective advertising campaigns, many of which feature well-known celebrities highly endorsing their products, their message has certainly received wide acceptance.

However, you have to remember that these products generally have not undergone the stringent testing to determine their effectiveness, and more importantly, they most likely have not been adequately tested for their safety. That is the key. Vitamins and nutritional supplements have not met the rigid requirements the Food and Drug Administration places on pharmaceutical companies prior to introducing a medication to society. We really don't know what the potential long-term consequences are of some of the herbs and nutritional supplements that are highly promoted. Taking these supplements without the consent and knowledge of your doctor could in the long run lead to health problems.

Let's review some of the most common vitamins, herbs, and nutritional supplements recommended to reduce your risk of developing coronary heart disease or further complications if you have been diagnosed with the disease.

Beta-carotene

Beta-carotene is an antioxidant that becomes vitamin A when metabolized in the body. Available data from several completed large-scale, randomized, interventional trials indicate that beta-carotene supplementation for periods of up to 12 years has no benefit in well-nourished populations on the incidence of coronary heart disease or the middle to late stages of cancer. There are several ongoing trials that are testing the possible long-term overall effect of beta-carotene supplementation in high-risk patients or individuals who have existing cancer or significant cardiovascular disease.

One study looking at beta-carotene is the Physicians Health Study, an ongoing study evaluating its impact on cardiovascular diseases and cancer. This study is monitored by doctors at the Harvard Medical School and involves over 20,000 U.S. physicians, and includes the dietary supplementation of beta-carotene. After 10 years, beta-carotene has not been shown to have any positive effect on the existence or prevention of cardiovascular disease or cancer.

In some older medical textbooks, a disease called "Bear Hunters" syndrome is described. It is the result of excessive ingestion of beta-carotene. It manifests as significant skin rashes, hair loss and sometimes liver inflammation. It is called Bear Hunters syndrome because it was observed in many Canadian and northern U.S. bear hunters, who often cooked and ate bear meat, which is rich in Vitamin A and is thus connected to beta-carotene. With both the Physicians Health Study and Bear Hunters syndrome in mind, it is not advisable to supplement your diet with beta-carotene except for that which is present in a multiple vitamin and a prudent (i.e., low fat or Mediterranean) diet.

Recommendation of beta-carotene supplements for prevention of coronary heart disease—**NO**, only that dosage which is present in a multiple vitamin.

Garlic

A common over-the-counter nutritional supplement that has been touted to lower total cholesterol and "maintain good cardiovascular health" is garlic. Considerable advertising and promotion of garlic supplementation has been targeted toward its contributions to cardiovascular wellness. On the basis of a number of new, well-designed, interventional controlled studies, there is increasingly less **evidence of cholesterol-lowering properties in garlic preparations**. A number of studies with very clear negative results have been published which demonstrate that garlic preparations are not useful for lowering LDL-cholesterol or total cholesterol concentrations. There have been no well-controlled studies examining the impact of garlic supplementation on the prevention of cardiovascular diseases. Therefore, at this time supplementing your diet with a garlic tablet is not recommended

Much of the advertising supporting garlic's role in lowering LDL-cholesterol or total cholesterol has come from manufacturers, suppliers, or sponsors of a particular garlic preparation.

In 1998, two European physicians, Drs. H. K. Berthold and T. Sudhop,[3] evaluated all of the available data from clinical studies concerning garlic supplementation on blood cholesterol levels as well as cardiovascular and cancer outcomes. As a result of their extensive evaluation of all of these studies, they concluded that garlic has no benefit on reducing blood cholesterol levels or reducing risk of cardiovascular disease or cancer. Yet despite this information, manufacturers of garlic supplements continue to saturate the airwaves with messages announcing the potentially positive aspects of taking garlic. This is not directed at singling out garlic. I am simply trying to show you that caution must be exercised when considering taking a nutritional supplement or herb for reducing cholesterol or reducing your risk of coronary heart disease.

Recommendation of garlic supplements regarding cholesterol levels—**NO**, there are no benefits from garlic supplements on reducing cholesterol levels or the risk of coronary heart disease.

Vitamin E

Vitamin E has been studied as a nutritional supplement for reducing the risk of cardiovascular events. Three large interventional trials of coronary heart disease patients supplementing their diet with 200 to 800 units of vitamin E have been conducted. **Unfortunately, the results are inconclusive.** One study called the

---

[3] Dr. H.K. Berthold and Dr. T. Sudhop: Garlic Preparations for the Prevention of Atherosclerosis; Current Opinion in Lipidology Vol. 9, pages 565- 569, 1998.

Cambridge Heart Antioxidant Study (CHAOS) found that people with coronary heart disease who took either 400 or 800 units of vitamin E per day had a 25% reduction in subsequent coronary events compared to the individuals taking a placebo. In addition, the benefit of vitamin E was the same in both groups—those taking 400 units and those who took 800 units. In a more recent study conducted in Canada called the Heart Outcomes Prevention Evaluation (HOPE), Study, the effect of taking vitamin E had no impact on coronary heart disease outcomes after 5 years of follow-up. This trial included 9,541 persons 55 years of age or older who had coronary heart disease, prior stroke, or diabetes. An additional interventional trial of vitamin E has also been negative.

There have been a few isolated reports in the medical literature indicating that people taking in excess of 2,500 units of vitamin E per day have increased bleeding tendencies including hemorrhagic stroke and intestinal bleeding. A few reports have also indicated mild increases in blood pressure with excessive vitamin E supplementation. Therefore, with regard to vitamin E, dosages of 400 units, or less, appear to be safe. Furthermore, since no reported adverse events have been identified from the three large interventional studies, one might consider taking no more than 400 units of vitamin E along with a prudent diet if you have coronary heart disease. It appears that the vitamin E should be of the natural form, which means it is extracted from soy beans, and this will be so indicated on the label. Since vitamin E is not absorbed on an empty stomach, it should be taken with food. (Actually, any vitamin supplement should be taken with food to maintain absorption.) You need not fear side effects at small doses (i.e., 400 units or less). Remember that one study (CHAOS) did demonstrate a clinical benefit. Obviously more research is required to determine whether vitamin E should be routinely prescribed or not prescribed for patients with coronary heart disease.

Recommendation of vitamin E supplements for prevention of coronary heart disease— MAYBE, more research is needed. However, in the meantime, small doses of vitamin E—400 units or less, will not produce adverse effects and may be of benefit.

Folic Acid (Folate)

Another vitamin that may be considered if you have coronary heart disease is folic acid. Folic acid is one of the B vitamins, B9 to be exact. It effectively reduces homocysteine, an amino acid intermediate found in the blood. (Remember, amino acids are the building blocks of protein. However, this discussion does not mean to imply that eating moderate amounts of protein leads to elevated levels of homocysteine. This is not true.) Elevated blood levels [concentrations greater than 12 micromoles per liter (mcmol/L)] of homocysteine have been associated with increased risk of coronary heart disease and stroke events in several observational trials. Basically, high levels of homocysteine have been detected in some patients with coronary heart disease, and it is therefore, considered a *risk factor*, not causally related.

Since the results of several observational studies have confirmed that high homocysteine is a risk factor, your doctor may recommend that you take a daily multiple vitamin containing 400 micrograms (mcg) of folic acid, particularly if your homocysteine level is higher than 12 mcmol/L. Your physician may recommend even more folic acid should the blood homocysteine concentration be markedly elevated (i.e., greater than 15 mcmol/L). Bear in mind however, that while it has been clearly demonstrated that folic acid reduces homocysteine, no good interventional or clinical trial of reduction in coronary heart disease or stroke with lowering homocysteine by folic acid supplementation has been conducted as of this writing.

Until such a study is conducted and completed which shows true cause and effect benefits of homocysteine and folic acid supplementation, we can glean some information from the Nurse's Health Study. This was a large study of nursing health care professionals in the United States that examined a number of potential cardiovascular risk factors relative to the occurrence of coronary heart disease. In a substudy (small group of the total number of participants) of the Nurse's Health Study, it was observed that nurses who supplemented their diets with 500 or more mcg of folic acid per day had less coronary heart disease. Homocysteine concentrations, however, were not measured in this study, although it was believed that the beneficial effect of folic acid was, in part, through lowering homocysteine. Since no side effects were observed with this amount of folic acid, you may consider supplementing your diet with folic acid (400 to 800 mcg daily). Again, no proven effectiveness has been demonstrated, but the suggestion is that folic acid may be beneficial, and therefore, you may be "stacking the deck" in your favor by taking it.

Recommendation of folic acid supplementation for the prevention of coronary heart disease—**MAYBE**, no proven effectiveness has been determined at this time. However, it may be beneficial taken in doses of 400 to 800 mcg daily (from a multivitamin).

Fiber

Fiber is a polysugar that makes up most of the structural component of plants. Fiber is indigestible. The most familiar source of fiber is bran, which is the covering of the seed within the inedible husk. Fiber may be classified as soluble or insoluble. Wheat bran or brown rice tends to be rich in insoluble fiber. Insoluble fiber has been linked with a healthy large intestine because it helps the large intestine absorb water and provides a bulky mass for it to push on, which prevents you from becoming constipated. Insoluble fiber helps in the prevention of constipation, hemorrhoids, and diverticulosis, and may also help to protect against colon cancer as well. However, this has not been proven adequately in controlled interventional studies.

Oat bran and rye tend to be rich in soluble fiber. Soluble fiber slows the movement of food through the stomach and upper digestive tract, which promotes the feeling of fullness and sometimes will stave off hunger. It also slows the absorption of sugar, which keeps blood sugar levels higher for longer periods of time, and therefore, fends off hunger. Soluble fiber has been shown in controlled interventional studies to lower total cholesterol and LDL-cholesterol levels. As you know, bile from the liver and gallbladder contains cholesterol, which is normally reabsorbed from the small intestine and recycled. Soluble fiber binds bile and prevents its recycling. This results in the loss of bile from the body. Therefore, the liver will remove cholesterol (i.e., LDL) from the blood to manufacture more bile. This in turn reduces the blood concentration of total cholesterol and LDL-cholesterol.

The American Heart Association recommends 20 to 25 grams of fiber per day for a person with coronary heart disease. An average size apple contains about 3.5 grams of fiber and a piece of whole wheat bread contains about 2 grams of fiber. Fiber can be supplemented to the body in the form of psyllium hydrophilic mucilloid (brand name Metamucil®). One tablespoon contains about 3.5 grams of fiber. A diet high in fiber or supplemented with psyllium hydrophilic mucilloid is an effective way of lowering plasma LDL-cholesterol concentrations. You can expect a 10% to 12% lowering of your blood LDL-cholesterol level with a daily ingestion of 20 grams of fiber. However, while fiber binds to bile, it also can bind certain minerals such as iron, calcium, and zinc and carry them out of the body, possibly leading to deficiencies. Therefore, should you decide to supplement your diet with fiber, it is a good idea to also take a multiple vitamin either two hours before, or several hours after, you take the fiber supplement (i.e., psyllium hydrophilic mucilloid—Metamucil).

Recommendation of fiber for coronary heart disease patients—**YES**, 20 to 25 grams per day accompanied by a multiple vitamin.

Flavonoids

Flavonoids occur naturally in most fruits, vegetables, tea, wine, and fruit juices. They are similar in many respects to vitamins. It has been observed in survey studies that people who consume beverages containing flavonoids (wine, tea, and fruit juice) have a lower incidence of coronary heart disease and stroke. However, no well-controlled interventional studies have demonstrated this conclusively. Moreover, the long-term consequences of chronic flavonoid ingestion are not understood. While high consumption of fruits and vegetables along with a modest intake of red wine (no more than 4 ounces per day) should be encouraged, it does not seem advisable at this point to make a recommendation for supplementing your diet with a capsule containing flavonoids.

Recommendation of flavonoid supplements for the prevention of coronary heart disease and stroke—NO, it is not advisable at this time to supplement your diet with a flavonoid tablet. Rather, increased consumption of flavonoid-rich vegetables and some fruits is encouraged.

Soy

Soy are products derived from the soybean, which belongs to the legume family. Soybeans contain all of the building blocks of protein (called amino acids) as well as iron, folic acid, calcium, potassium, and the B vitamins. Soybeans are the base of such foods as soy milk, soy nuts, tofu, and soy flour.

Soy products are low in saturated and total fat and high in fiber. Most soy products contain isoflavones which are a specific type of flavonoid (see earlier discussion of flavonoids in this chapter), that may help to prevent coronary heart disease. As stated in the October 25, 1999 issue of the *Detroit Free Press*, the Food & Drug Administration (FDA) agreed to allow manufacturers of soy products to advertise that they can help to lower LDL-cholesterol and prevent coronary heart disease when consumed as a part of a prudent diet. It is believed that the high isoflavone content of soy may actually increase the HDL-cholesterol and decrease the LDL-cholesterol concentration in the blood. The fiber content of soy will also help reduce the LDL-cholesterol concentration.

Soy products may also help minimize hot flashes experienced by some women during menopause. The isoflavones possess mild estrogen activity that may reduce these menopausal symptoms and promote bone strength.

The amount of soy protein required to promote beneficial effects on blood cholesterol levels is about 25 grams per day. This can be accomplished by drinking soy milk (I think the vanilla flavored soy milk is particularly good) instead of milk and using it in cereals, desserts, hot chocolate, or soups (tomato, bean, etc.). Soy milk can also be mixed into yogurts, pasta dishes, and tomato sauce. An eight-ounce glass of soy milk contains about eight grams of soy protein. Soy flour can be used as a substitute for flour in baked goods—just replace 25% of your regular flour with soy flour.

Recommendation of soy products for patients with coronary heart disease—YES, it is believed that soy products, used in combination with a prudent diet

can help to prevent further coronary heart disease complications by lowering LDL-cholesterol levels.

Conclusion

It is vitally important to discuss with your doctor any decision regarding nutritional supplements that you may be considering. There are many that have not been discussed in this book and therefore, you can assume that I do not recommend supplementing your diet with any of them; at least not at this time. Generally, nutritional supplements have not undergone the same stringent testing that pharmaceutical drugs have undergone. In addition, companies manufacturing these substances are not under the strict laws of the Food and Drug Administration as are prescription medications. Also, remember that long-term safety of many of these products has not been established.

Chapter 9
Other Important Considerations

The purpose of this chapter is to "tie up some loose ends." It will attempt to review an assortment of other issues not previously discussed in this book that may have relevance toward your personal contribution to reducing your risk of having additional complications from your coronary heart disease. Many of these issues have been highlighted from time to time by the media and some insight about their relationship to or value for reducing coronary heart disease complications would be helpful.

Alcohol

Alcohol consumption is a poignant issue for people with coronary heart disease. Benefits about its consumption for lowering risk of coronary heart disease are widely discussed by the media. As a coronary heart disease patient knowing the pros and cons of alcohol consumption is essential.

Modest alcohol intake—one 4-ounce glass of wine, or one 12 ounce bottle of beer or 1 to 1.5 ounces of spirits in a cocktail, per day has consistently been shown to reduce the risk of having a heart attack. It is believed that modest quantities of alcohol are beneficial, in part by reducing the chance of a clot forming in a coronary artery partially narrowed by cholesterol accumulation. Alcohol may also reduce the risk of developing cholesterol blockages (i.e., atherosclerosis) through raising HDL-cholesterol blood levels. Remember that HDLs are the scavenger lipoproteins that remove excess cholesterol from artery walls, thereby preventing it from accumulating. **Clinical studies also consistently show that increasing your alcohol intake beyond a modest amount does not provide additional insurance against coronary heart disease complications.** Remember that excessive or chronic alcohol intake predisposes you to several health hazards including accidental injury, liver disease, poor judgment, and some forms of cancer, such as pancreatic. It generally is not recommended to start drinking to lower your risk of coronary heart disease.

Wine seems to receive more attention than other forms of alcohol as a means of reducing risk of coronary heart disease. Red wine, in particular, has been hypothesized to be part of the basis for the so-called "French Paradox." The French Paradox is the low incidence of coronary heart disease and heart attacks among the French who consume high amounts of saturated fat and have high blood concentrations of LDL-cholesterol. The red wine is hypothesized to negate the detrimental effects of the saturated fat and contribute to the unexpectedly low incidence of coronary heart disease. However, this is just a theory and has not been proven in a controlled interventional clinical trial. It is simply an observation made from a few survey studies.

These studies suggest that red wine, primarily red wines made from the petite syrah grape, may have additional benefit in reducing coronary heart disease beyond its alcohol content. Red wine may prevent the oxidation of LDL. Red wine grapes (particularly syrah and petite syrah) contain high concentrations of flavonoids and flavonoids are potent antioxidants. Research studies have observed that if LDL becomes oxidized it is much more likely to deposit its cholesterol in the lining of arteries. Therefore, in theory, if you can reduce the oxidative capacity of the body thereby reducing the amount of LDL being oxidized, you should reduce the amount of cholesterol being deposited in the coronary artery walls. So, red wines may reduce the risk of coronary artery disease by both the alcohol (i.e., reduce the clotting activity of the blood and raising the HDL level) and flavonoid (reduced oxidation of LDL) content.

It is always dangerous to recommend alcohol intake as a way to reduce the risk of coronary heart disease. Acknowledging the possible benefit of drinking alcohol increases the prospect that people will justify consuming more than is beneficial, which can lead to devastating consequences. Keep in mind that alcohol's benefit in reducing coronary heart disease is in effect after only one conservative serving per day. In short, you reap red wine's benefits through one 4-ounce glass per day. Consuming more does not provide any added benefit. Should you be attempting to lose weight, alcoholic beverages, whether they are wine, spirits or beer, are quite high in calories and you must take that into consideration if you are on a weight reduction diet.

Again, in making this decision, you should consult your doctor and realize that the consequences of alcohol consumption are real. If you are a disciplined person and you have coronary heart disease, one glass of red wine per day, along with a prudent diet may reduce your risk of subsequent coronary heart disease events.

Coffee

Unfiltered coffee brews contain a substance called cafestol that raises blood triglyceride and total cholesterol concentrations in humans. This component is in particularly high amounts in commercial blends of arabica and robusta coffees. In addition, unfiltered coffee brews such as Scandinavian boiled coffee and Turkish coffee contain high amounts of cafestol. These unfiltered coffee preparations contain approximately 5 mg per cup. The majority of commercial coffees contain approximately 2 mg per cup. Controlled clinical studies have shown that for each 10 mg of cafestol, serum triglycerides are increased by 15% after eight to twelve weeks and LDL-cholesterol about 17%. Therefore, you can expect that two cups of filtered coffee per day would raise your LDL-cholesterol concentration about 6%. Decaffeinated coffees are relatively ineffective in raising LDL-cholesterol or triglyceride blood concentrations. If you are a regular coffee drinker, drinking decaffeinated coffee is another way in which you can help lower your LDL-cholesterol level. Lowering or eliminating caffeine may also help to reduce your blood pressure.

One cup of regular coffee per day is acceptable, after that, substitute *decaffeinated* coffee in place of regular coffee.

Aspirin

Aspirin is a drug that reduces pain, fever, and inflammation and also decreases the clotting ability of blood. This latter property can reduce the risk of a heart attack and death in people with coronary heart disease. The American College of Cardiology recommends that patients with coronary heart disease take a baby aspirin to an adult aspirin daily or every other day. The decision about the dosage will be made by your doctor. He, or she, will take into consideration the other medications you may be taking (i.e., blood thinners such as warfarin or clopidogrel) and your sensitivity to aspirin (some people may experience stomach upset from an adult aspirin). The strength of an adult aspirin is 325 mg, while a baby aspirin is 81 mg. Several controlled, interventional studies of aspirin intake have clearly shown a benefit. People with coronary heart disease who take an aspirin daily reduce their risk of having a coronary event by about 25% to 30% compared to those who do not take an aspirin daily.

As indicated, the benefit of taking aspirin is rooted in its ability to reduce the formation of blood clots. The platelet, which is a component found in blood, is involved with forming blood clots. As previously emphasized, coronary arteries that are narrowed due to cholesterol deposits are predisposed to blood clot formation, and therefore, heart attack. By taking an aspirin tablet daily, you reduce the chances of a blood clot that could form in the narrowed portion of a coronary artery.

In addition, aspirin *may* also be important in reducing the inflammation associated with the most fragile cholesterol blockages. The emphasis here is placed on *may*. As previously indicated, recent research has shown that cholesterol deposits or plaques in coronary arteries that are vulnerable to heart attack (those that are blocking the artery generally less than 50%) also have significant inflammation associated with them. Inflammation is the body's response to injury. It's actually one of the body's defense mechanisms. Since cholesterol accumulating in the lining of a coronary artery is an injurious situation, white blood cells, which offer defense to the body, tend to accumulate underneath the plaques and in the areas of the lining of the artery where cholesterol is located. These white blood cells cause inflammation by secreting chemical substances which breakdown the scar tissue in the cap surrounding the cholesterol making it thin and prone to breaking. Should the cap break open and expose the underlying cholesterol and inflammation to the blood, platelets will become active and form a clot which can completely block the artery and the flow of blood. Essentially, the blood clot plugs the artery and causes a heart attack. A beneficial effect of the white blood cells is their ability to engulf and consume the accumulating cholesterol.

Aspirin's cardiovascular benefit may therefore, be through reducing the risk of heart attack in two ways: (1) by lowering the chances of a blood clot forming and (2) by lowering the inflammation caused by white blood cells in the cholesterol plaques.

The aspirin one takes should be enteric coated. This is a hard, candy-like coating that prevents the aspirin from dissolving in the stomach thereby preventing stomach upset. An enteric coated adult, or baby aspirin, dissolves in the intestine and eliminates stomach upset.

People with a healthy heart and coronary arteries should not take aspirin to prevent a heart attack or stroke without their doctor's specific recommendation. This is because, by reducing the ability of the blood to clot, it increases the chance of bleeding. The point here is that taking aspirin isn't for everyone. Consult with your doctor before deciding to take aspirin to reduce your risk of having a heart attack.

Antibiotics

Since we have discussed the issue of inflammation in coronary heart disease, you should be reminded that one of the proposed ways that statins (cholesterol-lowering drugs) stabilize the atherosclerotic plaques (blockages) most likely to cause a heart attack is by reducing the inflammation in the plaques (Chapter 5). By doing this, the surrounding scar-cap thickens, rendering strength and stability to the plaque. It will be much less likely to rupture, leading to a blood clot forming and a subsequent heart attack.

Like statins and aspirin, antibiotics may also be useful in this regard. Antibiotics are drugs that destroy or suppress bacteria, and are widely used to prevent and treat infections. Recently, several **observational** studies have reported a higher prevalence of infective microorganisms (i.e., bacteria) among individuals who have had recent heart attacks compared to individuals without coronary heart disease. Of course, this does not prove or indicate that infection causes coronary heart disease or heart attack. Rather, this observation generates a hypothesis that infection may be involved and that antibiotics may be useful for reducing the risk of a coronary event.

Again, this is highly theoretical at this time. We don't know the answer yet. However, since it is a new theory, the press has written about it and may have given misleading information to the public. This theory is currently being tested in controlled, interventional studies which are looking at the impact of giving antibiotics versus a sugar pill to people with coronary heart disease and then monitoring them for coronary events. After several of these studies are completed, physicians may be able to make recommendations regarding antibiotics. Until then, we are dealing with a lot of "what ifs." Therefore, even though it is interesting to speculate on this issue, and while more discussion is likely to be reported by the media, it is highly premature to think that antibiotics may provide a clinical benefit in reducing the risk of heart attack. As a sidelight to this discussion, when considering antibiotics for minor problems (e.g., colds), we cannot overlook the effects of long-term use of them. They can make the body resistant to infections and may cause a person to develop infections that aren't easily cured. Antibiotics should only be taken when there is a clear indication for their use.

ACE Inhibitors

Another category of medicines that may have important beneficial effects for people with coronary heart disease is the ACE (angiotensin converting enzyme) inhibitors. As discussed in Chapter 2 these medicines are vasodilators which means that they relax the arteries and thereby increase their inner diameters. This reduces the pressure in the arteries caused by the blood pushing up against the inner wall. While these medicines are highly effective for lowering blood pressure and are the cornerstone of medical therapy for patients with congestive heart failure, they also have benefit for people with coronary heart disease. A recent controlled, interventional study (called the Heart Outcomes Prevention Evaluation or HOPE study; remember this study also found no clinical benefit from taking vitamin E) found reductions in cardiovascular deaths, myocardial infarctions, strokes and the need for heart bypass and angioplasty procedures among patients with coronary heart disease taking the ACE inhibitor, ramipril, versus those taking a placebo. **These benefits were independent of the blood**

pressure lowering effect of ramipril.

The investigators of this study speculated that these benefits were through stabilizing the coronary artery plaques most vulnerable to causing a heart attack. As has been emphasized, a major benefit of taking statin medicines (LDL-cholesterol lowering medicines) by patients with coronary heart disease is plaque stabilization. Whether some of the mechanisms for leading to atherosclerotic plaque stabilization by statins and ACE inhibitors are the same or not needs to be identified.

The HOPE trial is the first such study to demonstrate the benefits of ACE inhibitors on reducing coronary heart disease events and requires confirmation. However, the results are so encouraging that they should prompt you as a coronary heart disease patient to discuss the issue of taking an ACE inhibitor with your doctor. Chances are you may have read or heard about the benefit of ACE inhibitors and now being armed with the knowledge about them, you should have an informative discussion with your doctor as to their appropriateness.

Smoking

The correlation between cigarette and cigar smoking, and lung cancer and lung disease (e.g., emphysema), has been well known for years. Many people, still associate smoking with cancer and breathing disorders. However, this certainly is not the complete picture. Smoking is not just a major risk factor for the development of coronary heart disease and stroke, it is causal (like LDL-cholesterol) for the development of coronary heart disease. **Actually, smoking is the single most important preventable cause of death in the United States.** Smoking cessation reduces the risk of a coronary event by 30% among smokers with coronary heart disease. It is also important to recognize that smokers are not the only ones adversely affected by tobacco smoke. Environmental tobacco smoke (ETS) which is also referred to as passive smoke or second hand smoke, is a serious health hazard for nonsmokers, particularly children.

> Smoking increases the risk of a person with coronary heart disease to have a heart attack to two to three times more than that of a non-smoker.

Smoking or being exposed to environmental tobacco smoke temporarily increases the blood pressure because of the nicotine present in smoke. Nicotine increases the heart rate and causes the arteries of the arms and legs to constrict. Nicotine is not the only bad component of smoke. Carbon monoxide also is present in smoke and gets into the blood and reduces the oxygen available to the heart and other organs of the body. When cholesterol deposits build up on the inner walls of coronary arteries, smokers have a greater chance of developing a clot where the artery is narrowed because tobacco smoke can make the blood clot faster.

Smoking also reduces the levels of HDL-cholesterol, which is the "good" lipoprotein whose function is to remove excess cholesterol from the walls of arteries. Anything you can do to help maintain or increase your HDL-cholesterol level is extremely important, and quitting smoking is one such guarantee of your being able to do that. Other deleterious substances (e.g., tars) in cigarette smoke may also injure the linings of the coronary arteries and accelerate the accumulation of cholesterol in the walls.

No cigarettes are safe. Scientists have determined that smoking low-tar or low-nicotine cigarettes does not reduce the risk of coronary heart disease. **Many people who have switched to low-tar and low-nicotine cigarettes smoke more cigarettes and inhale them more deeply to make up for the reduced nicotine.** This can be potentially more harmful because through inhaling more deeply on low-tar and low-nicotine cigarettes, smokers take in more of the other harmful substances in cigarette smoke that increases the risk of coronary heart disease, and of course, lung cancer.

No matter how much or how long you have smoked, when you quit smoking your risk of heart attack drops. You cut your risk of death from a heart attack in half after just one year of quitting. However, studies show that, on average, it takes 15 to 20 years of smoking cessation to reduce your risk of heart attack to as low as someone who never smoked.

Nonetheless, it is obvious that one of the most important ways of reducing your risk of heart attack due to coronary heart disease, if you are a smoker, is to stop smoking immediately.

Exercise

A sedentary lifestyle (or physical inactivity) is a modifiable risk factor for coronary heart disease. Exercise is important for preserving or improving health, in general. Regular exercise helps to control and lower blood pressure and helps to prevent the development of obesity and diabetes mellitus. Additionally, regular aerobic exercise can assist in managing stress, reducing weight, improving one's body image, increasing HDL-cholesterol ("good" cholesterol), increasing physical strength, and strengthening the heart.

Aerobic exercise strengthens the heart by increasing collateral circulation in the heart muscle. If you recall from Chapter 3, by a process called angiogenesis, (development of new blood vessels) your heart is capable of compensating for areas of ischemia (reduced blood flow through the coronary arteries). Through regular aerobic exercise you help to promote this process. Aerobic exercise can stimulate expansion of nearby artery branches of a blocked coronary artery through the development of new tiny coronary artery branches that will carry more blood to the area of the heart muscle that has been affected by coronary heart disease. After you have been exercising regularly, this collateral circulation (new blood vessel development) will become well developed and the symptoms of angina may decrease or even disappear. In fact, because of the extra blood flow to the heart muscle, collateral circulation can help prevent the damage caused if a heart attack occurs. There is no better argument for incorporating some degree of exercise into your daily life.

Aerobic exercise is the type of exercise that allows for maximum uptake of oxygen. Brisk walking, jogging, cycling and swimming are all examples of exercise that allow for extensive uptake of oxygen into the body and its organs. This type of exercise is the opposite of anaerobic exercise where only small amounts of oxygen are taken up by the body (including the heart). An example of anaerobic exercise is weight lifting.

If you have coronary heart disease and plan to begin exercising regularly, you must first consult your doctor. Your doctor will determine if it is suitable for you to exercise and, if so, at what level of exercise. This is to make certain that the exercise will help you, not harm you. Aerobic exercise builds stamina, increases flexibility and strengthens the cardiovascular system, while anaerobic exercise (i.e., weight lifting) builds strength.

For coronary heart disease patients, aerobic exercise is preferred because it improves cardiovascular fitness and health (and promotes the development of collateral circulation). The intensity of a workout is easily identified by comparing your heart rate (i.e., pulse) during exercise to the **target exercise heart rate.** The target exercise heart rate is the heart rate you should achieve and maintain to receive the optimal cardiovascular benefit.

The target exercise heart rate is determined as follows:
220 - age X % = target exercise heart rate.

Percentages (%) for those with coronary heart disease, approved for exercise by their doctor are as follows:

60%   Beginner
70%   Intermediate
80%   Physically Fit

Once you have calculated your target exercise heart rate you then begin your aerobic exercise activity slowly (walking, stationary cycling, swimming, etc.) and increase the activity until your target exercise rate is achieved. Continue the activity and sustain the target exercise heart rate for 20 to 30 minutes. Should you begin to feel uncomfortable (i.e., light-headed, tired, short of breath), stop immediately and rest. Remember, it may take several weeks of gradually increasing your activity before you will comfortably and safely achieve your target exercise heart rate. As your fitness level increases, you can gradually increase your target exercise heart rate by increasing aerobic exercise intensity.

Your ultimate goal is to achieve and sustain for about 30 minutes a target exercise heart rate of: 220 - your age X 80%.

Your heart rate is measured by placing the first two fingers of your hand on the inside of the opposite wrist, or against the carotid artery in the neck (located on either side of the trachea, or wind-pipe). Hold your fingers on either location for 10 seconds and count the number of pulses. Multiply the number of pulses by six. Be sure to measure your heart rate while exercising. Should you stop exercising, your heart rate will drop and therefore, not be accurate.

Conclusion

Actively participating in the management of your coronary heart disease should focus primarily on lowering your LDL-cholesterol concentration, no matter what that level is, thereby minimizing the extent and threat of the cholesterol blockages in your coronary arteries from rupturing and causing a heart attack. Although your primary care doctor and cardiologist will play an active, important role in this endeavor through prescribing medications (e.g., statins) and a diet, you must also assume a major responsibility for your health. This means making lifestyle changes that will assist in lowering your LDL-cholesterol, as well as improving your overall health.

Discipline yourself to limit your alcohol intake to one drink per day (preferably red wine), quit smoking (if necessary) and take an aspirin daily if you have your doctor's approval. Additionally, exercise, even if you just start out by walking for 20 minutes, three times a week and then gradually increase the exercise to achieve an appropriate cardiovascular fitness level. **Remember that the "cure" for coronary heart disease resides in modifying your risk factors, and not with heart bypass surgery or angioplasty.**

Conclusion

You have been presented with a considerable amount of information regarding the definition, development, diagnosis, and treatment of coronary heart disease. I have attempted to describe these concepts relative to other cardiovascular diseases for the purpose of clarification and elimination of confusion. This information has been provided to you so that you can utilize it effectively and begin to take an active role in reducing your risk of encountering the problems associated with coronary heart disease—namely, heart attack, stroke, hospitalization, or sudden death. **Remember, knowledge is power and you have the power to control the destiny of your cardiovascular health.**

Before you can favorably impact the quality of your life and take control as a coronary heart disease patient, you must accept that much of what you have been led to believe about this disease and its treatment is obsolete and may not be completely accurate. It is important that you dispel the myths associated primarily with the treatment of this disease. If you have coronary heart disease with ponderous, angina-causing plaques (greater than 70%), you likely have many smaller plaques (less than 50%). These plaques are quite large under the surface of the artery lining where they cannot be visualized by coronary angiography. These plaques are far more likely to cause a heart attack than the plaques that are symptom-producing and treated by heart bypass surgery, angioplasty or the traditional medicines (e.g., nitrates, calcium channel blockers).

Remember the Common Misconceptions About Coronary Heart Disease. (Refer to Chapter 4 for additional information.)

Common Misconceptions about Coronary Heart Disease

▶ Heart bypass surgery and angioplasty cure, or partially cure, coronary heart disease.

▶ The degree of coronary blockages is a good indicator of the likelihood of a heart attack.

▶ Cardiovascular disease is primarily a man's disease.

▶ The only benefit of cholesterol-lowering medicines is reducing the blood cholesterol level.

▶ Cholesterol-lowering medicines (statins) are associated with serious side effects.

▶ Only high cholesterol levels are linked to coronary heart disease heart attack.

It is essential that you understand that heart bypass surgery and angioplasty do not cure coronary heart disease. These surgical procedures essentially alleviate the symptoms of the disease. The cure of the disease resides in managing your risk factors and most importantly reducing the blood concentration of LDL-cholesterol through diet, exercise, and a statin medication.

Compliance with this plan is obligatory if you want to reduce your chance of having additional coronary heart disease problems, a stroke, or death.

Once you accept this, you should be prepared to put yourself on aggressive risk factor modification and LDL-cholesterol-lowering programs. The first step is to begin taking a statin. Many people with coronary heart disease who have total cholesterol levels of 200 mg/dL or less (and LDL-cholesterol levels of 100 mg/dL or less) are not receiving a statin or engaging in an aggressive LDL-cholesterol-lowering lifestyle. They and/or their doctors may feel their LDL-cholesterol levels are acceptable. **This is not true.** If you have coronary heart disease, your total cholesterol or LDL-cholesterol concentrations are too high-whatever they are. A statin should be given to all patients with coronary heart disease for two reasons. The secondary reason is to lower the LDL-cholesterol, which as just mentioned, is too high regardless of your existing level. **However, the primary reason to take a statin is to stabilize the atherosclerotic plaques (blockages) that are most likely to cause a heart attack.**

Adopt the Mediterranean diet, which is a diet that has been proven in interventional studies to reduce the risk of heart attacks in patients with coronary heart disease. This is a diet that consists of about 40% of your calories from carbohydrates, 25% from protein, and 35% from fat. The fat should come from poly- and monounsaturated fats, which are found in cold water fish such as tuna and salmon and nuts such as almonds, walnuts, and peanuts. Monounsaturated fats tend to raise the HDL-cholesterol levels and prevent cholesterol from accumulating in the lining of arteries. Reduce dramatically your intake of all dairy products, animal meats and processed foods (cookies, cakes, and candies) which contain saturated fat and counteract the effectiveness of statins. A Mediterranean-type diet, with its low amounts of saturated fat, will allow the statin to work to its maximal ability.

It is also a good idea to drink 12 ounces of soy milk every day (the vanilla flavor is good), since it is a good source of protein. Put it on your cereal, mix it in your yogurt, or drink it instead of a glass of milk. The FDA has endorsed soy protein as an effective way to lower the LDL-cholesterol and reduce risk of coronary heart disease.

If you are overweight, you need to reduce the amount of food you're eating. Don't convince yourself that you have "low metabolism" or that your body just can't lose the weight. Be honest with yourself, and reduce your food consumption. It's just that simple. Your longevity, as well as the quality of your daily life, is closely linked to reaching and maintaining a proportionate, healthy body weight. *As you get older, you need less food, not more.* Therefore, you need to start altering your eating habits in an effort to reach and maintain an appropriate body weight. Drink a 10-ounce glass of water before each meal and snack to stave off excess hunger.

There are several other ways you can begin to reduce your risk of coronary heart disease complications. If you are smoker, **quit.** Smoking lowers your "good" cholesterol (HDL) and adversely affects your coronary arteries making them much more susceptible to cholesterol accumulation and blood clot formation. In short, smoking increases the chance that your existing blockages will lead to a heart attack

Exercise regularly. Aerobic exercise, such as walking, jogging, cycling, and swimming, allows the maximum uptake of oxygen. After you begin exercising regularly, your collateral circulation (new blood vessel development) will become better developed and the symptoms of angina may decrease, or even disappear. The extra blood flow to the heart muscle is of great benefit to you. It may save your life, should you suffer a heart attack.

It doesn't hurt for you to supplement your diet with 400 to 800 mcg of folic acid and 200 to 400 units of vitamin E daily. Several observational studies have indicated that those individuals who supplement their diets with 500 mcg, or more, of folic acid per day have a tendency toward less cardiovascular disease. One interventional study demonstrated that vitamin E supplements reduced coronary events in people with coronary heart disease. It is not recommended to take any more vitamin E or folic acid than what has been suggested. These vitamins should be taken with food to allow for appropriate absorption into the body.

Take one to two tablespoons of Metamucil® (psyllium hydrophillic mucilliod) every day. It is a good source of fiber and will reduce your LDL-cholesterol. Each tablespoon contains approximately 3.5 grams of fiber. Your total fiber intake per day from all nutritional sources should be 20 to 25 grams per day. Other sources of fiber include apples (3-4 grams), grain breads (2-3 grams per slice), whole grain cereals (4-5 grams) and fresh vegetables (carrots, celery, beans, peas).

Begin taking a baby or adult aspirin daily, unless you have a tendency to bleed or have some other medical condition like asthma, which can be complicated by aspirin. *Please talk to your doctor about the use of aspirin.* Aspirin reduces the clotting activity of blood and reduces the chance of a clot forming in a partially blocked coronary artery. Interventional studies have demonstrated that taking an aspirin reduces the chance of having or dying from a heart attack by 25% in those individuals who have coronary heart disease. The aspirin should be enteric coated. This is a hard, candy-like coating that prevents the aspirin from dissolving in the stomach, which could cause stomach upset.

If you can control your red wine consumption to only one glass per day, you may be helping yourself. However, remember, the benefit of red wine is in the first glass. One glass of red wine, particularly that made from syrah grapes, may mod-

Table 3. Summary of Treatments		
Proven to Lower the Risk of Heart Attack, Sudden Death, and the Need for Bypass Surgery or Angioplasty		
Treatment	**Risk Reduction**	**Major Mechanism(s)**
LDL-cholesterol lowering	40% to 45%	stabilize cholesterol plaques, and improve function of coronary arteries
Aspirin	25%	reduce the ability of blood to form clots
Exercise	10%	increase collateral heart circulation
Smoking cessation	30% (first 6 months)	improve function of coronary arteries and raise HDL-cholesterol
Beta blockers	15% to 20%	unknown, but probably lowering blood pressure, and reducing heart rate and workload on the heart
ACE inhibitors	25%-30%	reduce blood pressure and improve function of coronary arteries

estly raise your "good" cholesterol (HDL) blood level and reduce the clotting activity of your blood. The flavonoids (antioxidants) of the wine may also reduce the oxidation of your LDL, making it less likely to deposit its cholesterol in the linings of your coronary arteries. Drinking a second or third glass will not reduce your risk any further.

In addition, if you have already had a heart attack, you should probably take a beta-blocker as a way to reduce your heart rate, blood pressure and work load on the heart. You may, however, have special circumstances that would make taking a beta-blocker inppropriate or inadvisable. *You must talk to you doctor about taking a beta-blocker.* Other medications such as ACE inhibitors, nitrates, and calcium channel blockers may also be prescribed by your doctor.

It will help you retain the message of this book if you understand the information from the following acronym of *The ABC's of Coronary Heart Disease.*

A is for atherosclerosis
B is for bypass surgery and angioplasty
C is for cholesterol reduction
S is for stabilization of coronary plaques

The fundamental messages of this book revolve around the truth pertaining to the ABC's of coronary heart disease—**A**therosclerosis, **B**ypass surgery and angioplasty, **C**holesterol reduction, and **S**tabilization of coronary plaques. If you accept the evidence and if you follow the very basic guidelines for a healthier living that have been suggested in this book, you will go a long way toward increasing your chances of improving the quality of your daily life, for the rest of your life. I wish every reader of this book good health, and may God bless you and keep you healthy.

Epilogue

The twentieth century has seen a pandemic in cardiovascular diseases raging across the industrialized world. Significant cardiovascular disease research was initiated following World War II, and an enormous amount has been learned about the mechanisms, diagnosis, treatment and prevention of these diseases, particularly coronary heart disease. The past five years have generated important new information about coronary heart disease treatment and prevention. By virtue of what is now understood, it is realistic to establish the goal of ending the coronary heart disease pandemic by the third or fourth decade of the twenty-first century. While the medical profession will have the opportunity to play a key role in the realization of this goal, true success will only come about if society "takes charge" and adopts the measures that will end this pandemic. Success requires that the focus be on risk factor modification; primarily reduction of the blood concentration of LDL-cholesterol, and smoking cessation. While there is no absolute cure for existing coronary heart disease, amelioration is attainable through LDL-cholesterol reduction and smoking cessation, and will reduce the complications (and therefore, cost) associated with this disease. The real future, however, resides in primary prevention (prevention of the development of coronary heart disease). With the stout commitment of all of us, the battle against coronary heart disease can be won.

Glossary & Index

aneurysm

A balloon-like bulge that forms in an area of an artery where the wall is weakened or damaged, such as can occur with cholesterol accumulation. It is dangerous because it is susceptible to bursting, thereby causing intense bleeding (hemorrhaging) that can lead to death.

angina (also called angina pectoris)

A sudden severe pain or sensation of constriction over the front of the chest resulting from inadequate blood supply in the coronary arteries to the heart muscle (myocardium). The pain is usually increased with exercise and will subside with rest. It sometimes can spread to the jaw or the arms. It usually results from the narrowing by cholesterol accumulation in of one or more of the coronary arteries which supply the heart muscle with blood. It can be relieved by the use of drugs that either dilate (open up) the coronary arteries or reduce the force of the heart contraction.

angiography

A radiological technique used to demonstrate the pathways and configuration of blood vessels in various parts of the body. A radiopaque solution is injected into an artery that increases the x-ray contrast between the blood vessel and its surrounding tissues. After this injection, a number of x-rays are taken in rapid succession to follow the course of the blood. The technique is primarily used to show narrowing or cholesterol blockages of the arteries in the heart, i.e., coronary artery disease.

angiotensin-converting enzyme (ACE) inhibitors

Drugs that help to open up blood vessels (dilate) by blocking an enzyme called angiotensin-converting enzyme. They are used to treat high blood pressure and heart failure. They are particularly useful in treating high blood pressure among patients with diabetes mellitus. Examples include: captopril (Capoten), enalapril (Vasotec), lisinopril (Zestril, Prinivil), fosinopril (Monopril), benazepril (Lotensin), quinapril (Accupril), and ramipril (Altace).

aorta

The largest artery in the body. It originates in the left ventricle of the heart and conveys blood to the rest of the body. It is divided into three parts: (1) the ascending aorta passing upwards, backward to the right, and giving two branches to the heart called coronary arteries, (2) the aortic arch crossing to the left side giving major branches of arteries to the head and the arms, and (3) the descending aorta, passing through the chest cage and abdomen before terminating in the major arteries of the legs (i.e., iliac and femoral arteries).

aortic regurgitation

Back flow of blood from the aorta into the heart during the relaxation period of the heart. It is due to defects of the aortic valve and can result in problems as minor as palpitations to as serious as pulmonary edema and heart failure.

arteriosclerosis

An umbrella term covering several disease changes in medium and large-sized arteries. The most important is atherosclerosis which is accumulation of cholesterol and scar (fibrotic) tissue in the inner lining of an artery. The term is often used synonymously with atherosclerosis.

atherosclerosis

A form of arteriosclerosis in which cholesterol is deposited into the inner wall of medium and large-sized arteries. Over time, scarring begins to occur, above the cholesterol accumulation and this causes narrowing of the affected artery. Common sites are the aorta and arteries of the brain, heart, and legs. The disease increases with age and is sometimes referred to as "hardening of the arteries."

atrial fibrillation

A type of irregular heart beat characterized by fine, rapid contractions or twitchings of the atria or reservoir chambers of the heart. It causes an ineffective contraction of the atria, and therefore blood does not flow properly from the atria into the ventricles or pumping chambers of the heart. Atrial fibrillation is usually associated with underlying heart disease such as coronary artery disease, valve disease, or heart failure.

balloon angioplasty (technically, percutaneous transmural coronary angioplasty (PTCA)

Insertion of a catheter or tube into a coronary artery that has been narrowed by cholesterol deposits. A balloon is positioned at the tip of the catheter and is inflated at the site of the blockage causing the blockage to squeeze or press up against the blood vessel wall. When successful, this procedure allows for blood flow to increase. It is used to treat narrowed arteries of the legs, kidney and heart (coronary arteries).

beta-blockers

Drugs that are used to treat high blood pressure or coronary heart disease. Beta-blockers dilate (open up) blood vessels and lower blood pressure, and reduce the heart contraction force that lowers the workload of the heart. These drugs also slow the heart rate. Examples include: propranolol (Inderal), sotalol (Betapace), timolol (Blocadren), metaprolol (Lopressor, Toprol XL), atenolol (Tenormin), nadolol (Corgard), and acebutolol (Sectral).

bradycardia

A heart rate less than 50 beats per minute.

bypass surgery (technically, coronary artery bypass grafting surgery)

A surgical procedure used to treat coronary heart disease symptoms. It involves attaching a graft (internal mammary artery or saphenous vein) to the aorta and a site on a coronary artery just below an atherosclerotic plaque. It provides for normal blood flow past the atherosclerotic plaque or blockage.

calcium channel-blockers

Drugs that lower blood pressure through relaxing and opening up arteries. They are useful for treating hypertension (i.e., high blood pressure). Examples include: diltiazem (Cardizem), verapamil (Calan, Isoptin, Verelan), amlodipine (Norvasc), nifedipine (Porcardia, Adalat), felodipine (Plendil), nicardipine (Cardene), and isradipine (DynaCirc).

capillaries

The tiniest blood vessels in the body. They are characterized by having small openings in their walls, called pores, which allow oxygen and nutrients to leave and carbon dioxide and waste products from cells to enter. They are formed from branching of the tiniest arteries, called arterioles. Capillaries converge to form the smallest veins, called venules.

cardiac arrest

Complete stoppage of heart function.

cardiac catheterization

A diagnostic procedure in which a catheter (tube) is passed through the femoral (leg) or brachial (arm) artery to the heart. The catheter allows the doctor to measure pressures in the heart chambers. A radiopaque (dye) substance can also be injected through the catheter so that the presence of atherosclerotic plaques in the coronary arteries can be observed by x-ray.

cardiac markers
Specific proteins contained in heart cells that are released into the blood stream when heart cells die as a consequence of a heart attack. The proteins include: myoglobin, creatinine kinase-MB, and troponins T and I. They are detected in elevated concentrations in the blood of heart attack victims.

cardiac tamponade
A condition caused by fluid accumulating in the sac (pericardium) in the chest cavity that contains the heart. The fluid compresses the heart and restricts its ability to function. Cardiac tamponade is usually caused by trauma leading to bleeding from the heart or major blood vessel near the heart. It is usually fatal unless corrected by the removal of the fluid or blood.

cardiogenic shock
Severe heart failure resulting in inadequate pumping of blood to all organs of the body. It can be caused by heart valve dysfunction, heart attack, and/or cardiac tamponade. The blood pressure is extremely low and not sufficient to sustain life.

cardiomyopathy
A group of diseases of the heart muscle resulting in inadequate filling and pumping by the heart. It is characterized by heart failure and dysfunction. Some of the causes are heart attack, valve disease, and high blood pressure. The excess use of alcohol can also lead to cardiomyopathy. Sometimes the causes are unknown-this is referred to as idiopathic cardiomyopathy.

catheter
A long, narrow tube used in cardiac diagnostic and therapeutic (e.g., angioplasty) procedures. It is inserted into either an artery in the leg (femoral) or the arm (brachial) and advanced into the heart or coronary artery.

cholesterol
A type of fat which is an essential component of cell membranes and the precursor of bile and adrenocortical and sex hormone production. (An excessive amount in the arteries can cause atherosclerosis leading to coronary artery disease.) Cholesterol is found only in animals.

chylomicrons
A large lipoprotein in the blood that is manufactured by the small intestine and contains the fats obtained from the diet. Normally, chylomicrons are not present in the blood after a 10 to 12 hour fast. They are comprised mostly of triglyceride.

circulation
The movement of blood through the blood vessels (i.e., arteries, capillaries and veins).

collateral circulation
New and detoured circulation of the blood through smaller arteries that develop in the heart muscle as a result of exercise or because a main branch of the left or right coronary artery has been blocked off (i.e., heart attack).

congestive heart failure
A condition of several problems of the heart resulting in its inability to pump enough blood for the body's normal requirements. Causes include high blood pressure, loss of pumping ability by the heart due to heart attack, cardiomyopathy (idiopathic) and high blood pressure. It is one of the most common reasons for hospitalization in men and women over the age of 65. It is characterized by fluid retention in the lungs,

swelling of the feet and ankles, and enlargement of the heart.

coronary arteries

Two main arteries and their branches that supply the myocardium (heart muscle) with blood that provides the oxygen and nutrients required for normal function.

coronary artery disease

Atherosclerotic plaque (cholesterol blockages) within the inner linings of the coronary arteries. It is technically different than coronary heart disease, although the terms are commonly used inter-changeably.

coronary heart disease

Damage to the myocardium (heart muscle) resulting from heart attack (myocardial infarction) that occurred in a coronary artery containing athero-sclerotic plaque. It is the leading cause of morbidity and mortality is most westernized countries. It is also known as ischemic heart disease.

coronary occlusion

An obstruction (usually a blood clot) in a branch of one of the coronary arteries that hinders blood flow to a portion of the heart muscle. This part of the heart muscle dies because of reduced blood flow. Also called thrombosis or myocardial infarction.

C-reactive protein (CRP)

A protein found in the blood of people that have inflammation in their body. It tends to be in high concentration in the blood of people with inflam-matory diseases such as arthritis. It has recently been found to be elevated in the blood of people with coronary artery disease who have later had heart attacks.

culprit lesion

The cholesterol blockage, or plaque, in the coronary artery that breaks open and is responsible for a heart attack. The degree of vessel narrowing caused by a culprit lesion is usually less than 50%.

diabetes mellitus

A relatively common metabolic disorder in which sugar (carbohydrate) utilization is reduced. It is caused by an absolute deficiency of insulin (Type I) or by resistance to the effect of insulin (Type II). Of the 15 million Americans with diabetes, 90% have Type II. Patients with diabetes mellitus are at very high risk of developing coronary heart disease.

diaphoresis

The medical term for excessive sweating or perspiring. It is one of the symptoms of a heart attack.

diuretic

A drug, sometimes called a "water pill," that promotes excretion of urine. These drugs are useful in reducing swelling (or edema) in the ankles, feet,or lungs of patients with congestive heart failure. They are also useful for reducing blood pressure. Examples include three types: (1) Thiazides: chlorothiazide (Diuril), hydrochlorothiazide (Hyzaar, Dyazide, Maxzide, HydroDIURIL), indapamide (Lozol), (2) Potassium-Sparing: triamterene (Dyrenium), spironolactone (Aldactone), and amiloride (Midamor); (3) Loop Diuretics: furosemide (Lasix), ethacrynic acid (Edecrin), and bumetanide (Bumex).

echocardiogram (ECHO)

A heart test that gives a moving picture, or image, of the heart. It shows the motion of the valves and whether there is valve disease or not. A probe is placed on the chest that emits sound waves which bounce off the heart and back to a video screen.

electrocardiogram (ECG or EKG)

A diagnostic test for investigating the electrical activity of the heart. The test indicates whether the heartbeat is normal or not. Electrodes are placed on the chest, wrists, and ankles and a tracing of the heart's activity takes place over several minutes. Also referred to as EKG.

epidemic

A disease or disorder affecting many individuals throughout an area at the same time.

fasting lipid profile

Blood levels of total cholesterol, triglyceride, LDL-cholesterol, and HDL-cholesterol after fasting for 12 hours.

foam cells

macrophages residing in the inner lining of an artery that have engulfed large amounts of LDL and cholesterol. They are a major component of atherosclerotic plaques.

glucose

A simple sugar common in most plants and animals. It is the major source of energy for the body.

graft

A surgical procedure of implanting live tissue or the joining of tissues. For example, the surgical attaching of one open end of a saphenous vein to the aorta and the other end to a coronary artery. (This is referred to as coronary artery bypass grafting surgery.)

HDL-cholesterol

The cholesterol contained in high density lipoproteins (HDL), which are scavenger lipoproteins that remove excess cholesterol from the cells of the body, including the artery wall. It is commonly referred to as "good" cholesterol.

heart attack (also called myocardial infarction and coronary thrombosis)

It is the death of muscles cells of the heart occurring when oxygen and nutrients carried by the blood are abruptly stopped due to a coronary artery being completely blocked. It is usually preceded by attacks of chest pain or angina pectoris. The cardinal symptom is pain over the chest that does not subside with rest, but persists for several hours. The effects vary with the site and extent of the heart muscle involved. It may cause little bodily disturbance beyond a few days of tiredness or lead to heart failure, irregular heartbeats, cardiac arrest, or sudden death.

heart palpitations

These are irregular heartbeats. They may be caused by heart disease, excess intake of stimulants such as caffeine or smoking, anxiety, or nervousness, or a precipitous increase in exercise. They should be evaluated by a doctor to determine whether the cause is serious or not.

hemorrhage

Bleeding, especially a large loss of blood from a blood vessel.

Holter monitoring

A test allowing for recording the heartbeat over a 24 to 48 hour period while the individual keeps a diary of their activities. Electrodes are placed on the chest and connected to a special cassette recorder that is placed on the waist. The electrodes and recorder are maintained for a 24 to 48 hour period. The heartbeat is recorded over this period and abnormalities in the rhythm can be determined.

hypertension

Chronic elevation of the blood pressure defined as greater than 140/90 mmHg. Hypertension increases the risk of atherosclerosis, heart attack, congestive heart failure, kidney failure, and cerebral hemorrhaging (i.e., hemorrhagic stroke).

hypertriglyceridemia
Elevation of the blood level of triglycerides after a 12 hour fast. Defined as greater than 200 mg/dL.

hypotension
Abnormally low blood pressure.

insulin
A hormone produced and secreted by the pancreas. It is essential to the regulation of sugar (carbohydrate) and fat metabolism. It is also administered for the treatment of diabetes mellitus.

interventional study
A type of medical research study where the ability of a particular intervention (e.g., medicine, vitamin, surgical procedure) to affect an outcome (e.g., hypertension, hypertriglyceridemia, obesity) is evaluated. Participants of these studies are generally randomized to the active intervention or a control (e.g., placebo or sugar pill). These types of studies provide the highest standard for establishing cause and effect.

intima
The innermost layer, or lining, of an artery. It is the layer of the artery that makes direct contact with the blood.

ischemia
The lack of blood flow to an organ (i.e., heart or brain).

ketosis
A condition characterized by the body producing ketones. Ketones are fragments of fats that are potentially toxic. This condition occurs when sugar is not available to produce energy for the body, such as in diabetes or starvation. Ketosis also occurs in diets that are extremely high in protein and fat, with very little sugar (e.g., Atkins' diet).

LDL-cholesterol
The cholesterol contained in low density lipoproteins (LDL), which are the lipoproteins that deliver cholesterol to cells in the body, including those of the artery wall. It is commonly referred to as "bad" cholesterol.

lipid
The technical term for fat. The major lipids in blood include cholesterol, triglyceride, fatty acid, and phospholipid. Lipids are carried in the blood by packages or containers called lipoproteins.

lipid triad
The term used to describe the concentrations of one lipid and two lipoproteins in the blood: LDL-cholesterol, HDL-cholesterol, and triglyceride.

lipoproteins
Packages containing fat that are found in the bloodstream. Since fats (cholesterol and triglyceride) are similar to oil and blood is mostly water, fats must be contained in packages to be transported in the blood. These packages called lipoproteins are spherical in structure and are composed of a coat of protein surrounding the inner fat core. There are four major lipoprotein packages carrying all of the cholesterol and triglycerides in the bloodstream.

lumen
The space in the interior of a tubular structure such as an artery, vein, or intestine.

lymphocytes

A type of white blood cell that makes up a part of the body's immune (defense against disease or injury) system. They are found in high concentrations in the most fragile atherosclerotic plaques (cholesterol blockages), those that can rupture and lead to a heart attack.

macrophages

large white blood cells that engulf and digest foreign substances, such as bacteria abd oxidized LDL, in the bloodstream an tissues.

metabolism

The body's chemical processes and activities. Metabolism is divided into synthesis (building process) called anabolism, and degradation, called catabolism.

mg/dL

Milligrams per deciliter. The standard unit of measurement for a concentration, or level, of a substance in the blood.

mmHg

Millimeters of mercury. A standard unit of blood pressure measurement. Normal blood pressure is 120/70 mmHg.

morbidity

An adjective that describes an abnormal condition or complication that has resulted from a disease; also a diseased state.

myocardium

heart muscle.

myocyte

A muscle cell. A cardiac myocyte is one of millions of cells forming the heart.

myxoma

A benign tumor of the heart.

nitroglycerin

A drug (called a vasodilator) that relaxes coronary arteries (opens them up) and allows for increased blood flow. It is used to relieve angina attacks (chest discomfort).

observational study

See *survey study*.

ostium

A small opening, or entrance, into a hollow organ, such as a blood vessel. An example is the two ostia in the aorta which are the origins for the right and left coronary arteries.

pulmonary edema

A condition often associated with heart failure where the left ventricle of the heart does not pump blood adequately. This results in a "backup" of blood in the lungs causing increased pressure in the lung capillaries, and fluid (plasma) is forced out of the capillaries into the surrounding lung tissue. This fluid accumulation in the lungs impairs breathing.

statins (3- hydroxy-3-methylglutary/coenzyme A reductase inhibitors)

A class of medications that are highly effective in lowering the total cholesterol, particularly LDL-cholesterol. These drugs tend to help the liver remove LDL from the bloodstream, thereby reducing its concentration. Examples include: lovastatin (Mevacor), pravastatin (Pravachol), simvastatin (Zocor), fluvastatin (Lescol), atorvastatin (Lipitor), and cerivastatin (Baycol).

stress test (stress EKG)

A stress test is similar to a regular EKG except that it shows the heart's electrical response to exercise. Electrodes are attached to the chest and an individual is asked to walk or jog on a treadmill. Various degrees of exercise are achieved and the EKG records the heart's electrical response. Should a patient be unable to walk or jog on a treadmill, a stationary bicycle or an ergometer can be used. The test is used to determine the possible presence of coronary heart disease.

stroke

A sudden interruption of the blood supply to a portion of the brain which results in the death of brain cells followed by varying degrees of disability in speech, sight, understanding, or movement. About 15% of strokes are caused by a rupture of a brain artery or blood vessel (called hemorrhagic stroke), while the remainder are caused by atherosclerosis (called ischemic stroke).

sudden death

Death due to the sudden loss of the normal heart rhythm, or beat. It can be caused by coronary heart disease or malfunctioning of the conduction of the electrical impulses of the heart that generate the heartbeat.

survey (or observational) study

A common type of medical research study where one or more characteristics (e.g., body weight, blood pressure, garlic ingestion, smoking habits) of a group of people are monitored over a period of time and then related to a particular outcome (e.g., cancer, heart disease, diabetes mellitus). These studies are useful for establishing relationships among characteristics and outcomes. However, a relationship, even a strong one, does not indicate cause and effect. Generally, relationships that are identified by these studies are tested for accuracy and authenticity by interventional studies. Examples of survey, or observational, studies include epidemiologic, case-control, and cross-sectional studies.

syndrome

A collection of signs and symptoms associated with a morbidity or disease process. The collection of problems together constitute the actual picture of the disease or disorder. Congestive heart failure is an example of a syndrome that results from the inability of the heart to pump blood adequately (i.e., heart failure). The signs and symptoms associated with this syndrome include high blood pressure, disease of the heart muscle (cardiomyopathy), sometimes valve abnormalities, difficulty with breathing and fluid retention in the lungs and swelling in the feet and ankles.

thorax

The part of the body that exists between the neck and the abdomen. It is enclosed by the vertebral column, the ribs and the sternum and is separated from the abdomen by the diaphragm. The thorax is also known as the thoracic cage or chest. The lungs, heart, esophagus (tube connecting the mouth to the stomach), thymus gland, and part of the thyroid gland exist in the thorax.

thrombosis

The formation of a blood clot within a blood vessel, resulting in either partial or complete blockage of blood flow. The process is often initiated by blood contact with a partially blocked artery due to cholesterol accumulation. Thrombosis or the formation of a blood clot can occur within either an artery or a vein. When a blood clot forms in a blood vessel, breaks away and lodges in a smaller vessel where it then obstructs the flow of blood, it is called an embolus.

unstable angina

Angina or the sudden severe pain or sensation of constriction over the front of the chest that does not relinquish with rest. The onset is unpredictable. It usually signals that a heart attack is likely to occur.

urea

A waste product of cellular metabolism containing nitrogen. It is carried in the blood and excreted from the body as blood flows through the kidneys. It is a major component of urine.

VLDL-cholesterol

The cholesterol contained in very low density lipoproteins (VLDL). Only 10% or less of the total blood cholesterol is contained in this lipoprotein. While in the fasting state (i.e., no food or drink, other than water, for 10 to 12 hours) VLDL contain most of the blood's triglyceride.